Medical Ethics

Surviving on the
and Passing Exams

Daniel K. Sokol

Gillian Bergson

Series Editor

Ashley McKimm

À maman et papa – *elle est à vous cette chanson*

About the authors

Daniel Sokol is a researcher in Medical Ethics at Imperial College, London. He teaches the subject to doctors and medical students, and writes regularly on medical ethics in academic journals, magazines and newspapers. He has featured on TV and radio, and is a regular contributor to the International Herald Tribune, The Times, The Guardian, The Independent and the BBC. He lives in Oxford.

10 05674325

Gillian Bergson is currently a 5th year medical student at Oxford University and St Peter's College. She is completing her clinical training at the John Radcliffe Hospital and has a special interest in medical ethics.

About trauma

trauma is the magazine for medical students — produced by medical students. Formed by students four years ago it is distributed free in all UK medical schools four times each year. Our international edition is available in 22 countries worldwide from Belize to Zambia — making us the world's largest free distribution student magazine!!

All our stories are written by students about topics they want to read. The latest news, features and resources have helped make **trauma** one of the top sources for information among the medical community. Freshers, elective and careers supplements support the content of our main magazine. We also compile the UK's only list of 180 intercalated courses which are becoming an increasingly important part of the medical degree course.

Our unique rep structure means that we have a presence in each medical school across the UK and around the world. The 'trauma Team' of over 100 people help ensure copies reach students through the medical schools, libraries and student unions. We keep our team informed of the latest updates through our 'trauma Team Talk' email list.

Online we offer students the web version of **trauma** along with access to the '**trauma** Community'. Free student email accounts, discussion boards and scheduled chat help bring our readers from around the world together. We also help students publish their work online and offer revision resources.

Produced entirely by medical students in their free-time we're extremely proud of our achievements over the past four years. Our presence in all corners of the globe is proof of the enthusiasm, energy and fun of the '**trauma** team' and '**trauma**' magazine.

Check us out and get involved at ***www.traumaroom.com***

Foreword

I wish I'd had a textbook like this on medical ethics when I was a medical student back in the early 1960s. Indeed I wish it had been available later on in my medical career. Straightforward, legally aware and legally checked, reflective, often very funny, yet clearly committed to helping readers understand medical ethical issues in the context of their professional and legal obligations, this is a book that any medical student and indeed many doctors will find very helpful. Perhaps the most remarkable feature of the book is that it is written by students, one researching for a doctorate in medical ethics at Imperial College, the other a clinical medical student at Oxford. Their primary objective was to produce a readable and simple – but in no way simplistic – textbook for medical students who want to pass their now compulsory examinations in medical ethics and law. (It's now difficult to believe that it was only in the 1990s that this subject became part of the core curriculum that medical students must study, be examined on and pass). The authors have admirably succeeded in these objectives, covering each of the twelve components of the core curriculum in medical ethics and law that were drawn up by a consensus conference of teachers of the subject. Beyond these objectives they have also provided an interesting and well-informed account of ethical issues that not only any medical student but also many practising doctors are likely to find engaging and stimulating. That cannot be said of many student textbooks.

The book is fascinating throughout – but I was particularly impressed with the helpful chapters on passing ethics exams and on vulnerabilities of medical students and doctors. With regard to the latter, one issue worth reiterating in this preface is the continuing concern among medical students about what to do when they are asked/told to carry out procedures that they believe would be wrong for them to carry out, or where they are concerned that a doctor is behaving unethically. Reasoned discussion of ethical concerns should know no hierarchies and I can only wholeheartedly agree with the authors (a) in encouraging (courteous) courage among medical students to discuss any such concerns with their teachers – their concerns may often be allayed by such discussion; (b) in exhorting medical schools positively to encourage their medical students to discuss any ethical concerns they may have, and to have clearly defined procedures for pursuing any that are not resolved.

Consideration of medical ethics has moved a long way since my own days as a medical student when I was told that it basically boiled down to doing as my teachers did, and told me to do. Serious consideration of this fairly short book will help the student of medicine – undergraduate or postgraduate – not only to pass exams, but also to be a better doctor. It might even – dare I suggest it? – help the well established doctor, for whom exams are a thing of the past.

Raanan Gillon, retired GP and Emeritus Professor of Medical Ethics, Imperial College London.

Table of Contents

This won't hurt: understanding medical ethics and ethical theory

Medicine is a most difficult art to acquire. All the college can do is to teach the student principles, based on facts in science, and give him good methods of work. These simply start him in the right direction; they do not make him a good practitioner – that is his own affair. William Osler

A few words about this book

This textbook has been written specifically for medical students and doctors in the United Kingdom. Whatever your medical school or specialty, it contains all the material you need to practise medicine ethically and to pass your exams in medical ethics. It assumes no prior knowledge of medical ethics, law or moral philosophy and uses clear and simple language. At times – and at our peril – we have tried to inject a dose of humour into the text. There is, without doubt, a link between learning and humour, as proved by the amusing acronyms that medical students use as memory aids.

The book draws on the experience of past and present students, leading medical ethicists, current examiners, lawyers, patients, and doctors of various grades and specialties. As far as possible, we have used real-life cases and actual exam questions to illustrate our points, although at times hypothetical scenarios were chosen to clarify or emphasize certain ideas. The end result, we hope, is a textbook that is comprehensive, easy to read, and relevant to both doctors and medical students.

Although the textbook principally targets medical students, nearly all the material should be of interest and relevance to practising doctors. We hope that the doctors reading this book will forgive us for addressing them, from time to time, as medical students. Perhaps they will take comfort in the fact that even the great William Osler, at the height of his fame, considered himself a medical student!

Why bother with medical ethics?

Many medical students (and, indeed, many doctors) are sceptical of medical ethics. They think it boring, pointless or so obvious that only fools need study it formally. So why study medical ethics?

• To pass Finals (or the ethics station of the MRCP exam)

Medical ethics and law are now a **compulsory part of the medical curriculum** in the UK. In 1996, teachers of medical ethics and law in UK medical schools got together to draw up a list of core topics. These topics make up the curriculum which all medical schools are advised to follow.

This book covers the entire curriculum, with each section covered by a separate chapter (see appendix A). A full chapter is devoted to passing exams. In it, you will find past exam questions from different medical schools with 'perfect' answers, advice on how to analyse a medical ethics case, guidance on writing longer ethics essays and useful tips from current examiners detailing what they love and hate in medical ethics answers.

For doctors preparing for the MRCP's 'ethics and communication skills' station, this book explains the ethical principles and legal rules which you are required to know.

• To be a more ethical doctor

Although in the pre-clinical years, ethics may appear dry and abstract, it is, in fact, an applied discipline. As you venture into the wards and witness consultations, you will realise that medical ethics creeps into everyday practice (see boxed text). PRHOs in the past have often lamented their 'ethical ignorance' when confronted with moral problems. They simply did not know what to do in certain situations. Medical ethics can shed light on the moral problems you will inevitably face as a medical student and as a qualified doctor. Ethical awareness is an integral part of being a good doctor.

A GP from Oxford:

"Our daily ethical problems are frequent but mundane: do we tell a relative or friend who comes to the desk asking if their relative or friend has an appointment? Or whether the relative has arrived at the health centre, or even registered with the practice? If I ring to give a patient a result but their relative is out, what is it best to say? Saying there is a result but not giving the answer raises anxiety, saying nothing but asking them to get the patient to ring back raises suspicions. How truthful should you be when you don't know what's going on, when you've made a mistake, etc. and the perennial "how to balance cost to the NHS with benefit to the patient". Should you force someone to stop driving after one episode of a faint which you're pretty sure is unlikely to occur in a car?"

• To avoid being struck off

Each year, the General Medical Council receives thousands of complaints. Most of those relate to an ethical violation. Each year, dozens of doctors get struck off for unethical behaviour. It would be a shame to waste five or six years of hard work at medical school only to get struck off once you qualify! No doctor or medical student wants to appear on the front page of the Sun with superimposed devil horns. Comparisons with Harold Shipman are seldom flattering. Appendix B, entitled 'How to get struck off', lists common mistakes that will land you in hot water.

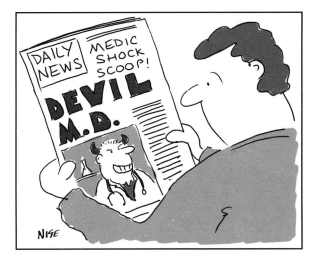

More than ever before, doctors must be able to justify their medical decisions to patients, colleagues and the courts. A sound knowledge of medical ethics and law will help you to formulate good justifications for your actions. A thorough reading and application of this book should prevent you from leaving the profession in disgrace.

Is medical ethics malodorous?

Although medical ethics is part of the core curriculum, the subject exudes a distinctly bad odour in the corridors and canteens of our hospitals and medical schools. Many medics frown upon medical ethics as an academic discipline. Yet, however much medics may moan about medical ethics, the truth is that medicine and morality cannot be separated. Medical ethics is as old as medicine itself. Until recently, however, medical ethics was not part of the medical curriculum. Medical students and junior doctors just learned ethics by observing their superiors. Now a discipline in its own right, medical ethics has a valuable role to play in the day-to-day practice of medicine. In this section, we address some of the common moans about medical ethics.

"Medical students have enough to learn as it is!"

Medical facts alone are worthless in practice. They become useful when they are applied to patients in particular circumstances. Medical ethics and law provide guidance on how and when to apply medical knowledge. The best doctors combine factual knowledge with an awareness of what is morally right and wrong, legal and illegal.

A junior hospital doctor:

"Working as a PRHO in paediatrics, paediatric surgery and adult medicine I am constantly surprised by how much I have used my training in ethics and law. It sounds like a cliché, but every day I come across situations where I have to make ethical decisions or know relevant medical law."[1]

"Medical ethics is a matter of opinion. There are no real answers"

A lot of medicine deals with known facts. All human cells, for example, have cytoplasm, but some things are less certain, such as the aetiology of certain cancers. The same is true of medical ethics. Many situations are obviously unethical. Everyone would agree that the murderous actions of Harold Shipman were morally wrong. Less obviously, if a consultant gets each of eight medical students to perform a digital rectal examination on a conscious cancer patient, without consent, most people would also condemn this as unethical. In many cases, then, there is an agreed right and wrong answer. The vast majority of ethical issues in everyday medicine are not a matter of opinion. They will have one (or more) right answers and many wrong answers. Only in difficult cases, such as deciding whether to abort a disabled fetus, will reasonable people disagree about which ethical path to adopt. Just as we don't consider medicine to be subjective because we don't yet know the causes of many psychiatric disorders, neither should we consider medical ethics to be subjective because some cases are difficult to resolve.

"Medical ethics is just common sense"

A lot of medical ethics is common sense. Obviously, most of the time doctors should be saving life rather than taking it and should promote the health of their patients. Nevertheless, some ethical problems are less clear. For example, consider this real case: a 33-year-old woman is heavily pregnant. Without a caesarean section, her baby will die and she will face a serious risk of death. She refuses the procedure on religious and cultural grounds. What is the right thing to do? Not all problems have common sense solutions. Some must be examined with a more structured approach, by identifying the conflict of values and principles, analysing the risks and benefits of each alternative, and arriving at a solution that can withstand criticism, even if not everyone agrees with it. As Voltaire said 'common sense is not so common'.

"Medical ethics is only a matter of law"

This is another common complaint: what's the point of studying medical ethics – all you need is law! So, in the case of the pregnant woman above, the ethical solution is to respect her refusal of treatment, since the law says so. Although knowledge of the law is important, it is not enough to resolve some ethical cases. Sometimes, the law is silent or unclear on an issue: Mary is a frail 80-year-old lady with inoperable lung cancer. She already knows about her grim prognosis. During a routine blood test, you realise she has liver involvement. Should you give Mary the results? The law provides little help in this case. Furthermore, what morality requires may be different from what the law requires. Imagine yourself in 1966, at a time when all abortion was illegal in Britain. If a traumatized 12-year-old girl, raped by a man with serious inheritable diseases, begged you to perform an abortion, you may have felt morally obliged to help her, although this was forbidden by the law. The law should play a role in the moral deliberations of doctors, but it doesn't always settle the moral issue.

"Medical ethicists are just busybodies who like criticizing doctors"

Medical ethics aims to analyse and promote the ethical practice of medicine. Most doctors work with laudable zeal and integrity. A few do not. Many doctors and medical students have stories about the ethically dubious actions of a colleague. Perhaps the colleague concealed information which you believed the patient had a right to know or maybe it was something more sinister. If taught properly, medical ethics provides tools that doctors and medical students can use to identify and resolve the ethical problems encountered in clinical practice. By the end of this book, you will hopefully find it easier to identify and analyse the ethical issues in a medical ethics case. Medical ethics is not the abstract and practically useless discipline that some think it is. Many North American hospitals now have full-time 'clinical ethicists' who help doctors resolve difficult moral cases. They are neither critics of the medical profession nor the 'ethics police', but an integral part of the health care team. Their primary role is to identify and clarify the moral issues in medicine and to suggest ways to address them.[2]

Ethical Theories at a Glance

You may already have heard a little about some of the ethical theories that are used to guide and justify ethical decisions. They include:

* Consequentialism
* Deontology (duty-based ethics)
* Virtue Ethics
* Principlism (the Four Principles approach)

Getting to grips with the main features of the different ethical theories can be daunting. To provide an insight into each of the main approaches, we have invited representatives of each ethical theory to comment on the case of Adam Zapple, a naïve young man who is tempted …

The case of Adam Zapple

Adam Zapple is feeling peckish. On his way home, he notices an elderly woman biting into an appetizing apple. Although only ten minutes away from his well stocked fridge, Adam considers mugging granny to steal her juicy-looking apple. Should he do so?

Over to our expert panel:

Kevin the Consequentialist: Well, this is an easy one! It's obvious that, on balance, mugging granny will cause more harm than good. Sure, Adam will enjoy the apple, but granny's misery will far outweigh his enjoyment. And let's not forget any bystanders who may get upset by the mugging. In fact, Adam himself might feel guilty afterwards, and get depressed. Now, if Adam was about to starve however …

Dan the Deontologist: It'd still be wrong, Kevin, you spawn of the devil! It's just wrong to beat up innocent people, whether it's to steal an apple or save your own life. There are some things people just shouldn't do!

Kevin the Consequentialist: Oh, so you'd rather die of hunger than steal an old lady's apple?

Dan the Deontologist: Definitely, stealing is wrong. Simple as that. What if everyone stole things whenever it suited them? No, I would kindly ask the lady...

Kevin the Consequentialist: to give you a new brain? No, seriously, why are some things 'just wrong'?

Dan: Too complicated for you, I'm afraid. Wait, let me work out the consequences ... (Dan mockingly takes out a calculator and presses on the keys)

Kevin: Go on, I'll try my best.

Dan: All right. One answer is that we should do – or not do – certain things because God said so in the Bible. 'Thou shalt not steal' is an example.

Kevin: Don't believe in God, sorry.

Dan: Fine. Have you ever heard of Kant?

Kevin: Sure, I love football!

Dan: No, the 18th century German deontologist philosopher!

Kevin: Oh. What's a deontologist?

Dan: Someone who believes that we should do things because we have duties or moral obligations to do them. We have a duty not to beat up innocent people or steal their property, for example, which is why Adam Zapple should not mug granny.

Kevin: Even if he's about to die of starvation and the granny is sitting on a barrel full of fresh apples?

Dan: Yes, stealing is wrong. Full stop.

Kevin: Weirdo.

Dan: Well, the World Medical Association has some deontological rules for doctors.

Kevin: Like what? 'Avoid deontology at all costs'.

Dan: No, 'The doctor shall not participate in the practice of torture or other forms of cruel, inhuman or degrading procedures, whatever the offence of which the victim of such procedures is suspected, accused or guilty, and whatever the victim's beliefs or motives, and in all situations, including armed conflict and civil strife'. That's a deontological statement.

Kevin: OK, it's a fair point but you should go out more.

Dan: Now, back to Kant.

Kevin: Oh good, I love football!

Dan: (expletives deleted) Kevin! Kant was a Christian, but he also believed that morality could be justified without invoking God. People, according to Kant, should follow the **Categorical Imperative**, which basically tells us what we should do.

Kevin: Wait, I know the answer: maximize happiness and minimize unhappiness!

Dan: Forget your consequentialist rubbish for a second! To satisfy the Categorical Imperative, Kant said we should follow two main formulas. The first is called the **Formula of Universal Law**. It tells us to 'act only on that maxim through which you can at the same time will that it should become a universal law'.

Kevin: You've lost me.

Dan: Basically, before you do something, ask yourself "Could I accept a world in which everyone did that?".

Kevin: I see. So, Adam should ask himself: "Could I accept a world in which everyone who was feeling peckish could beat up people to steal their food?"

Dan: Exactly. If the answer is 'no', then you shouldn't do it. It basically prevents people from being partial to themselves. The second formula is the Formula of Humanity. It tells us to always treat people as ends and never merely as a means.

Kevin: Uh, give me an example.

Dan: OK. When you take a taxi, for example, you're using the taxi driver as a means to your end: to get to your destination, but you're also paying him for it, so you're not using him only as a means. If you have a slave, however, then you are using him only as a means to your end. He's a tool which you can use as you wish. He has no choice in the matter.

Kevin: Ah. So Adam should not mug the granny because he would be using the granny merely as a means of getting the apple.

Dan: Precisely, but if he asked her and she consented, then it would be OK because he would be satisfying her wish as well as getting the apple.

Kevin: I understand. Deontology sounds fine in parts. After all, we're told as kids not to lie and not to steal and stuff, but I don't like the fact that consequences don't seem to matter much. Surely, if your life is at stake, then it's OK to lie?

Dan: Well, I don't like the fact that you're only concerned with consequences. If you're willing to break a promise if you think the consequences are better, for example, then how can people trust you?

Veronica the virtue theorist: Sorry, can I speak now? I think both your pet theories are wrong. Mugging granny for an apple is wrong not because of consequences or deontological rules, but because it's unkind and disrespectful. No virtuous person would do such an awful thing.

Dan: Sure, but what's a virtue?

Veronica: Good question. It's a character trait that's necessary for living well, such as courage, honesty, friendship, compassion, kindness and so on.

Kevin: Sounds a bit vague to me. This case is easy, but how do I know what a virtuous person would do in a really difficult ethical dilemma? What happens if two virtues clash with each other? If kindness requires me to be dishonest, for example? How do I decide which one trumps the other?

Paula the Principlist: Mmm, interesting. But let me try to break down Adam's case using the Four Principles.

Kevin: Oh gosh, here we go again. Good thing I always keep a pillow handy. I can snooze a little.

Dan: What are the Four Principles?

Paula: In a nutshell, there are four things you should and shouldn't do as an ethical person. First, you should respect the autonomy of other people. A person should be allowed to make his own choices, since only he knows what's best for him...unless he's not fit to make those choices, of course. Secondly, you shouldn't harm others, net harm that is, since almost every action can potentially cause harm. Thirdly, you should produce net benefit to certain people. And finally, you should be fair in offering your assistance, treat people equally, not discriminate. There, respect for autonomy, non-maleficence, beneficence and justice!

Dan: Sounds pretty good to me.

Paula the Principlist: Now, applying the principles to the case at hand, the principle of non-maleficence prevents us from causing net harm and here, clearly, Adam is causing more harm than good.

Kevin: Ah, I like this consequentialist thinking!

Paula: The principle of respect for autonomy, which tells us to respect people's freedom to make choices, also prevents him from mugging the old lady because she hasn't consented to this.

Dan: Sounds quite deontological to me. It reminds me of the Formula of Humanity: always treat people as an end and never only as a means.

Paula: Yes, it's a mixture really. It takes into account both consequences and moral rules, but it's not as black and white as Kevin or Dan's theories. It depends on the situation.

Paula and Veronica have provided only a brief introduction to Principlism (or the 'Four Principles' approach) and Virtue Ethics. We will say more on these approaches shortly. First, let us examine the reasons why ethical theories might be useful.

Do I really need to know that much about ethical theory?

For most non-philosophers, any talk of ethical theories will make them run a mile. However, a basic understanding of the main moral theories used in medical ethics can be useful for several reasons:

- It gives an **understanding** of where key concepts in medical ethics (such as consent and confidentiality) come from, and why they are important. Throughout the book, we will refer back to these theories to show how they have influenced many major 'rules' of medical ethics.

- It allows **flexibility**. The boundaries of medicine are constantly shifting, and ethical positions may need to be re-considered in the light of new developments. Take, for example, the current debate on abortion. Should we change the date limit for 'social' terminations to match the ever decreasing age at which premature babies can survive? Scientific progress regularly presents new ethical dilemmas. A sound knowledge of medical ethics provides tools to analyse these new problems.

- Ethical theories can be used to **justify** the ethical decisions that you make, either as a practising doctor or as a medical student sitting exams! An awareness of the main counter-arguments to your chosen solution can make your reasoning even stronger.

The case of Adam Zapple has hopefully provided you with an insight into these different theories. The main four theories of relevance – Consequentialism, Deontology, Virtue Ethics and Principlism – are summarised in the boxes below.

How to look clever with ethical theories

Consequentialism

In brief:
Only the **consequences** of an act are important.

The right action:
Is that which produces the **best consequences**.

Utilitarianism is the main consequentialist theory. It states that the right action is one that brings about the most utility. Utilitarians define 'utility' in different ways. For some, utility amounts to **pleasure** (hedonistic utilitarianism), for others it is **satisfying people's wishes** (preference utilitarianism) and for others still it is a **combination of desirable things**, such as beauty, love, friendship, pleasure and so on (pluralistic utilitarianism).

Of course, most of us believe consequences are important in deciding whether an act is right or wrong, but we think other things are important too, such as keeping promises. A consequentialist, however, believes that only consequences make an action right or wrong.

Main advantages:
- Consequences do matter for most of us.

- The theory doesn't discriminate between people. If the local dustbin man gets more utility from an act than David Beckham, then we ought to perform that act.

- In theory, deciding what to do is very simple: just work out which act produces the best consequences.

Main problems:

- Some actions seem to be wrong in themselves even if they lead to the best overall consequences. E.g. torturing an innocent child to save two other children.

- Maximising overall happiness may be unjust to certain individuals (such as the tortured child!).

- Calculating good and bad consequences can be very difficult. Actual outcomes may be different from the intended or probable outcomes.

- How can happiness or pleasure be measured? Right now, are you happier than I am? (probably not, since you're reading this!). How can you compare the happiness of different people?

- The theory is too demanding. Instead of watching our favourite TV show, we should be helping the poor in Africa or persuading all our friends to become utilitarians. It is unreasonable to demand that people maximise overall welfare all the time.

Deontology (duty-based ethics)

In brief:
Deontological theories identify various **duties** and rights. A duty is a **moral obligation** that a person has towards himself or others beings (e.g. *the duty not to steal*).

The **consequences** of the act are **not considered**. It is the *act itself* which determines whether it is right or wrong.

e.g. if stealing is morally wrong, then you should not steal, no matter how much good might result from your theft.

The right action:
Following morally required rules or principles.

Kant's **categorical imperative** gives some guidance on how to act in practice.

There are two important formulations of this:

1) Act only in such a way that you would be happy for it to become a universal law (Formula of Universal Law).

2) Treat people as ends in themselves, never just as means (Formula of Humanity).

Main advantages:
- Most of us believe that there are some things we should or shouldn't do, whatever the consequences.

- It upholds the dignity and intrinsic value of the individual.

Main problems:
- For most of us, consequences do matter, even if they are not everything!

- The nature of duties is not clearly specified. Do we have a duty not to lie? If so, how can we convincingly show this?

- What should we do when duties conflict?

Consider these two deontological duties
1. Do not lie.
2. Do not kill innocent people.

Now imagine a patient who is recovering from a heart attack and whose blood pressure is, at present, highly unstable. You get a phone call and are told that his wife of 40 years has died in a car accident on her way to the hospital. The patient asks you a question that can only be answered by telling him that his wife is dead. Should you lie?

If you tell the truth (and respect rule 1), you will most probably cause another heart attack (violating rule 2). This is the deontologist's nightmare!

This point is partly addressed by the philosopher William Ross, who introduced the idea of *prima facie* duties: when duties conflict, you need to judge which is the most important duty in the particular case.[3]

Virtue Ethics

In brief:
The **moral character** of the person performing the act is the important factor in assessing right and wrong.

The right action:
Is what a **virtuous person** would do in the circumstances.

Virtues are **attitudes that promote human flourishing** (e.g. courage, kindness, patience, charity, compassion, modesty).

Main advantages:
* Intuitively, it seems right to consider moral character in assessing right and wrong.

* Provides an explanation of why we act differently towards loved ones (by appealing to virtues such as friendship and loyalty, for example).

* Provides us with a richer moral vocabulary (e.g. benevolence, honesty, wisdom, compassion, and so on).

* In theory, what we ought to do is simple: do what a virtuous person would do!

Main problems:
* What are the virtues? It is not clear which traits of character should count as virtues.

* How do we know what a virtuous person would do if there is no defined set of virtues to guide us?

* The virtues may reflect the values of a particular society at a given time. If this is true, what counts as a virtue will vary over time and from culture to culture.

* More philosophically, why is it a good thing to have particular virtues? Why should I bother to be virtuous? The answer might refer to another ethical theory, such as utilitarianism or deontology. Virtue theory might need another ethical theory to make sense.

Principlism (originated by Tom Beauchamp and James Childress)[4]

In brief:

People should consider four *prima facie* principles when making decisions about ethics. These are:

- **Respect for autonomy** – the obligation to respect the decision-making capacities of autonomous agents.

- **Beneficence** – the obligation to provide net benefit to the patient.

- **Non-Maleficence** – the obligation to avoid causing net harm.

- **Justice** – the obligation to be fair in the distribution of health care resources.

Note: A *prima facie* moral obligation is one that should always be acted upon, unless it conflicts with another principle.

The right action:

The Four Principles are a starting point in the analysis of ethics cases. They don't provide solutions to ethical problems. You will need to **apply** the principles in a particular context and then **balance** them. See chapter 14 for details on applying the Four Principles.

Main advantages:

- Everyone agrees that the Four Principles are morally desirable.

- Provides a checklist for ethical decision making.

- Flexible – not as rigid as consequentialism and deontology.

- Easy to understand. Arguably easier to use in the clinical setting than other moral theories.

> **Main problems:**
> - No overarching moral theory binds the principles: where do the principles come from? Note that some see this as an advantage (see section below for details).
>
> - What should we do when conflicts arise between principles? There is no hierarchy within the principles.
>
> - The principles do not provide a solution to ethical problems, merely a framework with which to analyse them.
>
> - The principles can be interpreted and prioritised differently within different countries and cultures. The principle of respect for autonomy may not be given the same prominence in Outer Mongolia than in the UK.
>
> - Scope – to whom or to what do we owe the moral obligations reflected in the principles? Does the principle of non-maleficence apply to a fetus, for example?

For our purposes, the most important ethical theory to get to grips with is *Principlism*. Despite its deficiencies, we consider the approach well-suited to the practical needs of medical students and healthcare professionals. In this book, we frequently use the Four Principles approach when discussing ethics cases.

Why is Principlism a useful approach?

- The Four Principles approach is **compatible with a range of moral theories**. The independence of the Four Principles from any underlying moral theory is sometimes criticised as unsystematic. However, it is also an advantage. **Everyone agrees on the value and relevance** of these principles to ethical decision making. They transcend national, religious, cultural and philosophical barriers.

- Raanan Gillon describes the Four Principles as 'the four moral nucleotides that constitute moral DNA' arguing that alone or in combination, these principles are capable of **'explaining and justifying all the substantive and universalisable moral norms of health care ethics** and possibly also of ethics generally'.[5]

- The Four Principles are popular with students as they provide a straightforward tool with which to approach and analyse ethics cases.

- From the Four Principles, we can derive more specific, action-guiding rules (e.g. *obtain consent, respect confidentiality, be honest*), as will be shown in the next chapter.

In the exam section of the book, we will show how to use the Four Principles to analyse a medical ethics case. Like any methodological tool, the Four Principles can be used dreadfully by some and with great insight by others. Instruction and practice should place you in the latter category!

Understanding the Four Principles

Respect for autonomy

Respect the patient's right to make his own decisions about his life. Provide adequate information to allow informed decision making.

Example: The face of Kevin the Consequentialist has, for many years, been graced by an unsightly mole. As his long-suffering GP, you have suggested on several occasions that he have it removed. Kevin, however, has grown fond of this feature. He thinks it rather fetching. He therefore refuses all treatment, and you respect his wishes.

Recently however, the size and texture of the mole have begun to change and you are concerned that it might be cancerous. You try to impress upon Kevin the potential seriousness of not removing the mole. You give him all the information he needs to make an autonomous decision, based on true beliefs and an understanding of the situation. But Kevin, eager to maintain his desired cosmetic appearance, considers the risks worthwhile, and he elects to keep his hairy mole. Although you disagree, the principle of respect for autonomy requires you to respect Kevin's wishes.

Beneficence

Do good to your patients. Act in their best interests.

Example: Kevin the Consequentialist returns to your surgery for yet another consultation about his haemorrhoids. As he gets up to leave, he begins to experience crushing central chest pain and collapses by the door. You are worried that he may be having a heart attack and consider your options.

You don't really like Kevin that much but you remember the principle of beneficence – that as a doctor you should do good for your patients. As this man is having a heart attack in your consulting room, you concede that you ought to help him. You therefore call an ambulance for Kevin, and give him some GTN.

Non-Maleficence

Avoid causing net harm to patients (balance the likely harms of a potential treatment against its likely benefits). In every procedure, there is a risk of harm. In an appendicectomy, for example, the surgeon cuts someone's belly open, which in normal circumstances is highly undesirable. This means that if doctors were told to 'cause no harm', they would do nothing! The important thing is not to cause *net* harm. The likely benefits of an appendicectomy clearly outweigh the likely harms of the procedure.

Example: Kevin the Consequentialist survives his heart attack, but he is now furious. He blames your receptionist for causing the attack by wearing such a revealing blouse. In the weeks that follow, he becomes increasingly unpleasant towards you, turning up at the surgery daily to show you that he is still alive, "despite your best efforts" as he puts it.

You become increasingly irritated by Kevin and, on the brink of despair, you consider putting a strong laxative in his coffee to teach him a lesson. However, as you reach for the bottle, you remember the principle of non-maleficence. You abandon your idea, and wish him a good day.

Justice

Probably the most complex of the four principles. In short, the fair adjudication between competing claims, or not discriminating unfairly. There are various types of justice e.g. distributive (giving people their fair share), retributive (giving people their fair punishment), rights-based (respecting people's rights) and legal justice (acting according to the law). Some people equate justice with equality. Equality certainly has something to do with justice, but there is more to justice than mere equality. After all, it is possible to treat lots of people equally and terribly!

Example: Kevin the Consequentialist and Veronica the Virtue Theorist both present to your surgery seeking advice about painful in-growing toenails. You are happy to treat Veronica, who has always been a model of politeness and gratitude, the perfect patient in your eyes.

Kevin the consequentialist, on the other hand, is an odious man, who causes you great stress on a daily basis. Your gut reaction is not to treat him. However, you remember the principle of justice. As both patients have the same medical problem and can benefit equally from the treatment, you offer them the same treatment.

Your understanding of the basics of ethical theory, and in particular of the Four Principles approach should, at this stage, be much clearer than it was at the start of the chapter. Medical ethics, however, is more than the straightforward application of ethical theories. The discipline requires you to come up with good arguments for and against your position.

What is an argument?

An argument is a set of claims consisting of **premises** and a **conclusion**. The premises are intended to convince us that the conclusion is true.

Example: "Why couldn't I steal the apple from granny? She was sitting on a huge barrel of apples and she didn't *say* that she wanted to keep the apple!"

Comment: Adam Zapple is trying to convince us that he was justified in taking granny's apple by offering two premises: 1) that she had lots of apples anyway and 2) that she didn't object verbally. The argument is weak since the premises do not lead convincingly to the conclusion.

What is the difference between a *valid* and a *sound* argument?

In a valid argument, **the premises lead logically to the conclusion**. So, **if the premises are true, then the conclusion *must* be true.** It is impossible for the conclusion to be false if the premises are true.

Note that an argument can be valid even though the premises are false. What makes an argument valid is the **logical connection between the premises and the conclusion**.

Example of a valid argument:

If medical ethics is boring, then I'll eat my hat
Medical ethics is boring,
Therefore, I'll eat my hat

This is a valid argument, even though the premise that medical ethics is boring is obviously false! It is valid, but not *sound*. If medical ethics was actually boring, the argument would be sound.

A sound argument, therefore, is **a) valid** and **b) made up of true premises.**

What is a logical fallacy?

A fallacy is an argument that often seems plausible on the surface but that is actually wrong if you look a little closer. A logical fallacy is a **mistake in the logical relation between an argument's conclusion and its premises.** Identifying a logical fallacy is an important skill in argumentation and pretty darn impressive if you can identify it by name! There are dozens of different fallacies, but here are a few which you can spot everyday on TV, radio and in the newspapers:

* *Inductive fallacy of overgeneralization* – making a **broad generalization from a small sample.**

Example: Since *some* people don't want to know the truth about their illness, this means that all people don't want to know the truth about it.

* *The no-true-Scotsman fallacy* – rejecting a good counter-argument by **shifting the meaning of words.**

Example:
A: No Scotsman likes to mix haggis in his porridge!
B: But Lachlan MacDonald loves haggis in his porridge! He eats it three times a day. On Sundays, he even puts porridge in his haggis.
A: Ah, yes, but no *true* Scotsman likes to mix haggis in his porridge.

- *Appeal to authority* – Professor John Smith says that the moon is made of boursin (with a hint of herbs). John Smith is a world expert on the moon, therefore the moon is indeed made of boursin (with a hint of herbs). **The fact that an authority says X, does not *logically* entail that X is correct.** The authority might be wrong, his area of expertise might be elsewhere, or he may have been drunk or joking when uttering the statement! It is better to use independent arguments to support a position, not just the testimony of others.

Example: "Forget antihistamines, you should definitely buy that oil of earthworm lotion for your wasp sting; Sokol and Bergson recommend it!"

- *Ad hominem fallacy* – **attacking the source of the argument** instead of the argument itself.

Example: "How can Sokol say that doctors should be honest and trustworthy! With his receding hairline and booming voice, his risible glasses and decrepit bike, can we really take what he says seriously?"

- *Bifurcation* – **claiming that only two alternatives exist,** even though there are more.

Example: "If granny won't give me the apple, the only other option is to steal it!"

Recommended reading: Weston A. *A rulebook for arguments*. 2nd ed. Indianapolis: Hackett Publishing Company, 1992.[6]

Armed with our knowledge of ethical theory and argumentation, we will now turn our attention to specific areas of medical ethics and law covered by the Core Curriculum.

In the next chapter, we begin by looking at Informed Consent and Refusal of Treatment. It is probably the most important chapter in the book. Its contents represent the bread and butter of a doctor's ethical life. The chapter will illustrate the importance of the principle of respect for autonomy and the circumstances in which patient autonomy may sometimes be challenged.

Summary

A knowledge of medical ethics and law can help you:
* Be a better doctor.
* Pass your medical ethics exams.
* Avoid getting struck off the register.

Moral theories such as consequentialism, deontology, virtue theory and, in particular, principlism can be useful tools in the analysis of medical ethics cases.

We consider the Four Principles approach to be the most useful for medical students and healthcare professionals, although some philosophically-inclined medical ethicists may disagree. These principles are independent of, and to some extent compatible with, other ethical theories. They are universally accepted across national and cultural boundaries.

The 4 *prima facie* principles are:
* Respect for Autonomy
* Beneficence
* Non-maleficence
* Justice

Medical ethics requires you to come up with good arguments to justify your position.

References

1. Baxter C, Brennan M, Coldicott Y. *The practical guide to medical ethics & law for junior doctors and medical students*. Cheshire: Alden Group, 2002.

2. Sokol D, Benn P. Fresh insight, or rank nonsense? *Hospital Doctor* 2004:34.

3. Ross W. *The right and the good*. Oxford: Oxford University Press, 1930.

4. Beauchamp T, Childress J. *Principles of Biomedical Ethics*. 5th ed. Oxford: Oxford University Press, 2001.

5. Gillon R. Ethics needs principles – four can encompass the rest – and respect for autonomy should be "first among equals". *Journal of Medical Ethics* 2003;29(5):307-312.

6. Weston A. *A rulebook for arguments*. 2nd ed. Indianapolis: Hackett Publishing Company, 1992.

The bread and butter of a doctor's ethical life: informed consent and refusal of treatment

What is autonomy?

In the philosophical literature, barrels of ink have been spilt over the precise meaning of autonomy. For our purposes, however, autonomy refers to **people's ability to make rational choices based on their own beliefs and values, free from the controlling influence of others.** When Adam Zapple threatens to kick granny in the teeth if she refuses to hand over her apple, he is not respecting her autonomy. She doesn't have much choice in the matter. The fear of Adam's kung-fu kick in her shiny new dentures forces her to give away her apple against her will. Forcing people to do things is not respecting their autonomy.

Some animals appear to make choices but few people would claim that they are autonomous. They don't have the mental capacity to make rational decisions based on their own values. Autonomy, then, is more than merely choice. It is **informed, rational choice.**

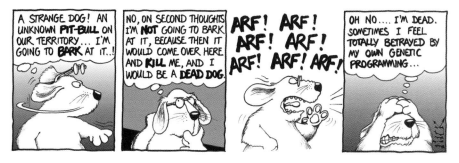

To make an autonomous decision, two things are needed:

1. **Freedom from undue influence**

2. **Mental capacity to make rational decisions**

Autonomy is not an all-or-nothing affair. It is a matter of degree. Usually, a 16-year-old is more autonomous than a 5-year-old, although a 5-year-old is still autonomous to some degree.

The autonomy continuum

No autonomy — — a little autonomy — — substantial autonomy — — full autonomy
this book   *a young child*   *most adults*   *Divine beings?*

No mortal is fully autonomous. There are always things we don't know (including the future). We should therefore respect the autonomy of substantially autonomous persons.

Why is respecting autonomy a good thing?

Kevin the Consequentialist would claim that respecting people's autonomy generally makes people happier than not respecting their autonomy. For this reason, respecting the autonomy of others should be encouraged (unless this harms others). After all, most of us want to make our own decisions, even if we may occasionally make bad ones.

Respecting a patient's autonomy is also more likely to ensure that net benefit is offered (principle of beneficence). **What constitutes 'benefit' varies in part from person to person:** a mastectomy for Mrs Smith might be beneficial, but for Mrs Jones it might be so horrible that she would rather not have the operation. **People are generally the best judges of what is in their best interests.** The principles of respect for autonomy and beneficence are thus not entirely separate. Knowing what people want forms part of knowing what is best for them.

Dan the Deontologist would allude to Kant, and say that not respecting people's autonomy is treating people merely as a means, and not also as an end, thus violating the principle of humanity. An essential part of respecting people is respecting their views and their ability to make personal choices. If we fail to do this, we are imposing our own views on them and preventing them from making autonomous choices.

So, in sum, respecting people's autonomy is good because:

a) it is likely to make people happier.

b) it shows respect for people's values and their decision-making ability.

What is the relevance of this to doctors and medicine?

In practice, respecting a patient's autonomy requires the doctor to:

- **Obtain informed consent.** Asking people for permission before you do things to them and giving them relevant information is respecting their autonomy. To make an autonomous decision, people must have enough information to make a choice which represents their true beliefs. If I consent to an appendicectomy believing that I only need to swallow a pill, I'm not making a sufficiently autonomous decision. I'm making an important decision based on factually incorrect information. Your duty, as a doctor, would be to **share any relevant information** to allow me to make a reasoned and informed choice. Respecting patient autonomy is the underlying reason for obtaining patient consent.

- **Respect patients' privacy and keep promises.** People rely on your confidentiality to run their lives. No one's going to tell you about their genital warts if you're going to post the fact on your website and tell your friends about them over lunch.

- **Not deceive patients.** This could take many forms, not just lying. Intentionally evading questions, using ambiguous language or even withholding information can be deceptive. Deceiving your patients will lead them to make decisions based on incorrect or insufficient information.

- **Help patients make decisions, if asked.** Not only can you respect their autonomy, but you can also enhance it. As long as you don't impose your views too vigorously, there is no reason why you should not offer your advice to patients.

- **Communicate effectively.** Patients must understand what is happening to them. Giving a patient all the relevant information about his impending appendicectomy is useless if you give it to him in Popoloca (unless the patient speaks this Mexican language, of course). Remember that, for some patients, medical jargon is as obscure as Popoloca, so try to avoid using recondite, polysemic or sesquipedalian words. Give patients the opportunity to talk and ask questions.

Vocabulary list:

recondite = out of the way or little known
polysemic = having many meanings
sesquipedalian = having lots of syllables

Note: use straightforward language when talking to patients

Should doctors *always* respect patient autonomy?

Remember that respect for autonomy is a *prima facie* principle. This means that it is not absolute, and that it can be trumped by overriding obligations.

- You don't need to obtain informed consent in an **emergency**, when a patient is in critical condition, for example. The reasoning behind this is that saving the patient's life takes priority when there is not enough time to obtain informed consent, or when the patient is unable to give consent.

Note: This applies when the patient is brought to hospital in a critical condition or, during an operation, when the surgeon discovers something life-threatening or so serious that it needs to be dealt with immediately. It does not apply when a competent patient has repeatedly refused a procedure, and then falls unconscious! You cannot just wait until a sick patient becomes unconscious and then perform a procedure on the basis of an emergency. A patient's valid consent or refusal of treatment does not vanish with his loss of consciousness.

True story:
A 33-year-old African woman is heavily pregnant in hospital. Without a caesarean section, her baby will die and she too will face a significant risk of death in labour. She refuses the operation on religious and cultural grounds. The doctors wait until she loses consciousness and then perform the caesarean section.

Verdict: Although highly distressing, the doctors should have respected the patient's refusal of treatment, even if there was a risk of death to both her and her unborn baby. The doctors did not have consent to perform the procedure on the patient, whether the patient was conscious or unconscious. Note also that the fetus has no legal status.

- You don't need to obtain informed consent when the **patient is not substantially autonomous** (e.g. very young children, certain psychiatric patients, or patients with severe learning difficulties). There are criteria for deciding whether a patient is sufficiently competent to consent.

- Sometimes, respecting a patient's autonomy will entail disrespecting other people's autonomy, including your own. If a patient wants you to amputate both his arms and legs so that he can enter the Paralympics, you are under no obligation to accept his request. If you discover that your patient's petechiae and conjunctival haemorrhaging are symptoms of the Ebola virus, you should disclose this to the relevant authorities on the grounds of **public health**. See the section on confidentiality (chapter 4) for more on this.

What's the big deal about consent?

Every day, as a doctor or medical student working with patients, you will need to obtain consent. It is therefore vital that you familiarise yourself thoroughly with the ethics and law regarding consent. It is not rocket science but, as the medical insurance companies will tell you, many medics fail to understand the purpose of consent or what is required to obtain it properly. Consent, in short, is more than a signature at the bottom of a consent form to get you off the hook in case of litigation.

What is consent?

The BMA defines consent as the **'patient's voluntary agreement to treatment, examination or other aspects of health care'.**[1] Consent can be given either explicitly or tacitly.

Explicit consent:

* In writing, e.g. signing a consent form.

* Orally, e.g. "I consent to this procedure".

Tacit (non-verbal) **consent,** e.g. opening mouth for tongue inspection.

Obtaining consent is ethically and legally required before any procedure or treatment is started on a competent, adult patient. As we saw earlier, it is a form of respecting autonomy.

> **Know your law:**
> - **Competent adults (i.e. 18 or over) can refuse *any* medical treatment,** including withdrawing current treatment, even if this entails certain death (this includes Jehovah's Witnesses who refuse blood transfusions).
>
> - An adult is **presumed competent** unless there is good evidence to the contrary.
>
> - **For incompetent patients, doctors should act in their best interests.** No one, even a next of kin or a court of law, can give or refuse consent on behalf of an incompetent adult. The doctor should act in the best interests of the patient. Nevertheless, it is good practice to consult relatives or friends, as they may provide an idea of what is in the best interests of the patient. They may know what the patient would have wanted in the circumstances, for example, or they may know the values dear to the patient.

Why is consent important?

Consent is important because:

- It is a good indication that the patient's autonomy has been respected. It allows patients to make their own decisions.

- If valid, consent acts as a pretty good guarantee that the patient has not been coerced into accepting a procedure.

- Patients are more likely to be helpful and cooperative if they actually want the treatment. In colonial times, Western doctors forcibly treated some African villagers with various drugs. One major problem with many of the health projects was that the locals failed to comply with the treatment regimes because they didn't want to be treated in the first place!

- You can be sued for battery or negligence if you fail to obtain consent properly! (see box below)

What is battery?
If a doctor (or medical student) touches a patient without consent, this constitutes **battery.** The patient can sue the medic.

What is negligence?
For a doctor to be considered **negligent,** the patient would need to prove that

a) the doctor had an obligation to care for the patient.

b) the doctor **did not provide an appropriate level of care,** as judged by a 'responsible body of medical people skilled in that particular art' (this is known as the **Bolam test**). The 'appropriate level of care' is judged in relation to your rank (i.e. if you're a PRHO, you'll be expected to be a competent PRHO, not a competent consultant), but if a competent PRHO would have asked someone more senior for help and you didn't, then you can be accused of not providing an 'appropriate level of care'.

c) the doctor **harmed the patient** (in contrast to 'battery', where no harm is necessary to be charged). This can be physical or psychological harm.

So, if you fail to warn a patient of a reasonable risk of a procedure and the risk happens, you can be sued for negligence *as long as the patient can prove that they would have declined the procedure had they known about the risk.* If they can prove this, then your omission to mention the risk is directly responsible for the patient's injuries and c), 'the doctor harmed the patient', is satisfied.

Reasons why a doctor may be found negligent include: a) failure to make a correct diagnosis b) failure to treat c) failure to warn of the risks of a procedure.

In practice – the importance of taking good notes

Good medical notes are important for two main reasons:

1. They **ensure that patients are treated effectively and appropriately** by providing information to all members of the healthcare team.

2. They **provide an objective record of a patient's care** that could be used in court in case of complaint.

The Medical Protection Society comments that 'the quality of care that a doctor has provided will, to a large extent, be **assessed by the standard of the notes** which form the foundation of the doctor's defence. Notes which are **inaccurate, illegible, inadequate or simply missing** will make most claims indefensible. Even if you have done nothing wrong in terms of clinical care, it is extremely hard to defend the claim unless you have medical records to prove it. **The courts are inclined to believe the patient's memory,** as it was probably a one-off experience for them, as opposed to that of the doctor who is recalling one of many similar consultations often many years later.'

> **True story:**
> A GP was called by a mother who was worried about her two-year-old daughter. The daughter was lethargic and had a high temperature. The GP made a home visit, examined the child and told the mother that it was probably flu but that she should call again if her daughter's condition got worse. He heard nothing more until the following morning, when the hospital informed him that the child had died of meningitis.
>
> The GP received a claim for clinical negligence. The notes were examined but he had made no record of the discussion or of the advice he offered. The claim centred on the mother's belief that she had not been told to call the GP if the child's condition deteriorated and that she was unaware that the situation could have been serious. As there was no record of the discussion, the claim was considered to be indefensible and an out of court settlement was agreed.

What are good notes?

For clinical and legal reasons, taking good notes is a vital part of a doctor's everyday work. Good notes should:

- Report the **relevant history.**

- Report the **relevant clinical findings.**

- Report the **investigations arranged** and the (provisional) **diagnosis.**

- Document the **decisions made,** including the drugs or treatment prescribed.

- Document the **information given** to patients.

- Include signed **consent forms** and **details of discussions** with the patient, including any advice given to the patient.

- Report **patient progress.**

- Note **referrals** and provisions for **follow-up.**

- Be **clear, legible and avoid ambiguity** (including in the use of abbreviations).

"The patient lives at home with his mother, father, and pet turtle, who is presently enrolled in day care three times a week." (courtesy of the MPS)

- **Identify the patient** on each page.

- Be **signed with date and time** and written in **permanent ink.**

- **Not contain offensive comments.** Remember that patients can legally ask to consult their notes, and so can the courts.

"I've met the patient, the wife, his children and the pet rabbit. Of the lot of them, the rabbit is the most intelligent"

"Exam of genitalia reveals that he is circus sized" (courtesy of the MPS)

Valid consent

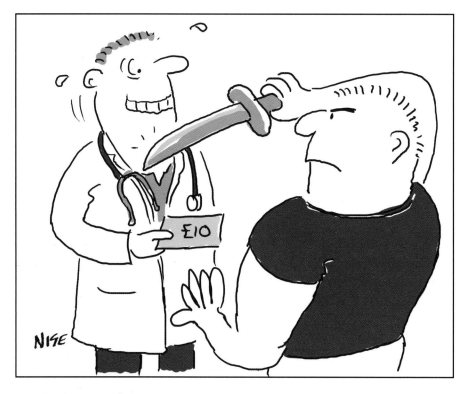

If an irate Mike Tyson, wielding a razor-sharp machete, asks you for £10, you don't really have much choice in the matter. Most competent, non-suicidal people would gladly hand over the £10. Although we would consent to giving him the money, the consent would not be valid, since we would be under considerable pressure to do so. Deep down, we probably don't want to give him £10. Less drastically, a patient who consents to a scrotal examination when surrounded by several consultants and half a dozen medical students is also under undue pressure to consent. He is likely to be intimidated by the throng of medics surrounding him, and might feel that his care would suffer if he refused. So, for consent to be valid, the patient must be **relatively free from pressure**. We say 'relatively' because everyone is under some pressure, however slight, to choose certain options. Think about your choice of medical school: were you not influenced by your parents, your friends, your school, or even the league tables?

What are the requirements for obtaining valid consent?

- The patient must be **competent**.

- The patient must **understand and believe** what he is consenting to. The procedure must be explained in a clear manner. The doctor must *ask questions* to ensure that the patient a) understands the situation b) believes what he is being told.

- The patient must be given **enough information** to weigh up the pros and cons and make an informed choice. This includes answers to the following questions:

  What is the purpose of the procedure?
  What does it entail?
  What are the likely and possible side-effects?
  What are the alternatives?
  What happens if nothing is done?

This means that **the doctor responsible for obtaining consent must be familiar with the treatment or procedure**. You can't obtain consent for coronary artery bypass grafting (CABG) or a highly complex operation if you don't understand it yourself! If unsure, ask someone more knowledgeable to obtain consent instead.

- The patient must be able to refuse.

- The patient must give consent voluntarily, relatively free from pressure.

- There cannot be too large a time delay between obtaining consent and the procedure itself ("...but yes, you *did* consent to this operation Mrs Smith, remember, February 1962?"). If there is a considerable time delay, the doctor should check with the patient that the consent still holds.

- The consent is specific to a treatment or procedure (i.e. the consent has a certain scope). So, if I validly consent to an appendicectomy, I also consent to the surgeon opening my belly with a scalpel. This falls within the scope of my consent. If however, the surgeon discovers something unrelated to the appendicectomy, then he does not have consent to fix it. He must obtain consent for that specific procedure once the appendicectomy is done, unless it is immediately life-threatening, of course, in which case it constitutes an emergency.

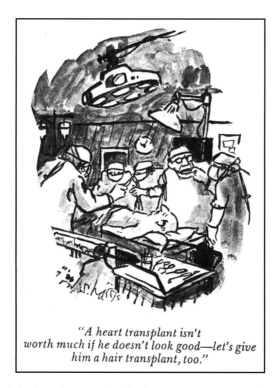

"A heart transplant isn't worth much if he doesn't look good—let's give him a hair transplant, too."

From the above, it is clear that a *patient's signature on a consent form is not, in itself, sufficient to prove that valid consent has been obtained.*

The myth of 'fully informed' consent

We often hear people talk of 'fully informed' consent. This is a misleading phrase. Doctors can't possibly tell the patient *everything* there is to know about a procedure, such as the type of suturing which will be used for example. This would most certainly confuse patients, as well as being tedious and time-consuming. The phrase 'adequately informed' consent is preferable. Doctors should provide enough information for patients to make an informed decision.

Remember that **different patients may want different amounts of information**. It is a doctor's duty to find out, through questioning, how much a particular patient wants to know. A patient may be given too much information! At a minimum, however, doctors should provide **enough basic information to allow patients to make an informed decision.**

According to the GMC, doctors should, if appropriate, provide:

- **Details** of the diagnosis and prognosis (including what is likely to happen if treatment is refused).

- **Uncertainties** about the diagnosis and the options for further tests before treatment.

- Different **options** for treating or managing the condition, including the option to do nothing.

- The **purpose** of the procedure, including what it entails, and what the patient is likely to experience during and after the procedure in terms of side-effects.

- How the condition (and side-effects) will be **monitored**.

- The **name of the doctor in charge** of the treatment and, if appropriate, the name of the senior doctors in the team.

- A **reminder** that patients can change their minds at any time and can seek a second opinion.[2]

True story:
In 1997, the singer Julie Andrews (of *Mary Poppins* and the *Sound of Music*) underwent an operation to remove non-cancerous throat nodules. After the operation, Andrews could no longer sing professionally. The surgeons failed to inform her of the small chance of losing her singing voice. Andrews sued the two doctors. The lawsuit was settled out of court.

Lesson: Use your nut! If you perform a procedure on Pavarotti's vocal cords or a pianist's hands, you should offer to give more information regarding possible side-effects than usual. A pianist (or surgeon) may view a 1/1000 chance of complications affecting finger joint movement very differently to a postman.

On a related point, you may not want to disclose a 1/1000 chance of a mild headache, but you should definitely mention a 1/1000 chance of quadriplegia or death.

In short:

- Use your common sense

- Mention very serious side-effects even if they have a low probability of occurring

- Don't mention very mild side-effects even if they have a higher probability of occurring

Thoughts on the value of moles– interpreting 'best interests'

True story:
A surgeon was successfully sued for removing a patient's mole when performing an operation to extract two wisdom teeth. The patient complained that he hadn't consented to the removal of the mole. This is an example of a doctor exceeding the scope of consent...and proof that people's idea of 'best interests' may be very different from our own!

The true story above shows how **people's idea of what is in their best interests varies from person to person**. Of course, most of us want good (or better) health, but many others things are important too. Our values, beliefs, and aims in life all play a role in deciding what we consider a 'good' life. The patient who sued the mole-hating surgeon obviously valued that part of his anatomy more than most. Perhaps the mole was the key to the patient's romantic success or perhaps the mole reminded him of his recently departed grandmother whose– admittedly unusual– last wish was for her grandson to keep the mole. This is why it's essential, when making a judgement about someone else's best interests, to **find out what sorts of things are important to them.**

There is a tendency for doctors to equate best interests with what is medically best. The medical component of 'best interests' is certainly important, but there are other considerations too. After all, it is the patient, not the doctor, who will live with the consequences of his decision. The doctor should therefore think of the concept of 'best interests' with an open mind.

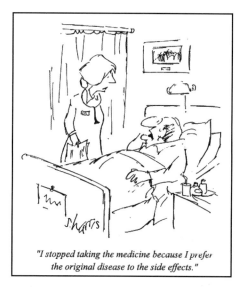

"I stopped taking the medicine because I prefer the original disease to the side effects."

Competence to consent

Competence and autonomy are related concepts. 'The criteria of the autonomous person and of the competent person are strikingly similar' as Beauchamp and Childress comment.[3] **Competence, however, is specific to a particular task,** whereas autonomy refers to a person's level of competence more generally. A child can be competent enough to decide whether to tie his shoelaces, for example, but not competent enough to decide whether to undergo heart surgery. Competence, in short, is **task-specific**. Also remember that patients can be more competent at certain times than others. Patients may be tired, confused or under considerable stress. If a patient's competence fluctuates or is temporarily affected (after a general anaesthetic, for example), it is best to wait until it returns to 'normal' before obtaining consent, except in an emergency.

Also, the fact that a patient has a psychiatric disorder doesn't necessarily mean that he cannot make *some* decisions. It depends on the nature of the disorder, as well as the type of decision to be made.

Patients are competent to consent as long as they understand the information, can weigh up the pros and cons, and, finally, if they actually believe that what you tell them is true. Some delusional patients, for example, may refuse to believe that you are telling the truth, although they may understand the situation perfectly. Other patients may believe you but not have the brain power to understand what's really going on.

What are advance directives?
An advance directive is a type of advance statement, which **indicates a refusal of treatment** in the future. It allows a person, who is currently competent, to have a degree of control over their treatment at some future time when they might no longer be competent.

What is the law on advance directives?
An advance refusal of treatment is *legally binding* if:

1. The adult who made the directive was competent at the time.

2. The patient had sufficient, accurate information to make an informed decision.

3. What is written in the directive applies to the particular circumstances.

4. The patient was not under any undue influence when making the directive.

Important: In the case of genuine doubt over the validity of an advance directive, you should provide life-saving treatment. If time permits, you should seek a court declaration.

Pros and cons of advance directives

Pros:

• Allows competent patients to exercise their autonomy.

• It may give patients, relatives and the medical team some peace of mind.

• It may lower costs to the NHS by avoiding expensive end-of-life treatment.

Cons:

• There may be difficulties in interpreting advance directives. Does the description on the written statement match the patient's medical condition?

• People can change their minds without changing the advance directive.

• It is not easy for people to imagine what it is like to be very ill.

• Patients can make advance directives based on insufficient or incorrect information.

Consent for studying and teaching

Patients *volunteer* to be part of medical teaching. Their consent is therefore required. Remember that patients are doing you a favour by allowing themselves to be scrutinised and palpated by curious medical students! Even if you're only sitting in on a GP consultation, you must make sure that the patient is comfortable with this. Ideally, the doctor should obtain consent in private, *before the consultation*. Patients should not feel under any pressure to consent, so a reassurance that a refusal will not alter their treatment is good practice. They should also be reminded that they may change their mind at any time without penalty.

• When a medical student is about to perform a procedure, it is also good practice for the doctor to inform the patient that a medical student will be carrying out the procedure. The doctor should add that the student has been trained and will be closely supervised.

William Osler (1849-1919)– a good role model
Osler was probably the most famous doctor of his day. He was renowned for his clinical skill, his love of teaching, his brilliance of character, and for insisting that medical students go on to the wards to learn medicine. Much of his advice remains as fresh today as it was then. Read Osler and you are guaranteed to become a better doctor!

A selection of quotes:
"A physician who treats himself has a fool for a patient"

"The physician needs a clear head and a kind heart"

"Care more particularly for the individual patient than for the special features of the disease"

"The practice of medicine is an art, based on science"

"To have striven, to have made an effort, to have been true to certain ideals– this alone is worth the struggle"

For further reading:
* Osler W. *Aphorisms from his bedside teachings and writings*. New York: Henry Schuman, Inc, 1950.

* Osler W. *A way of life*. New York, London: Paul B. Hoeber Inc, 1937.

* Osler W. *Aequanimitas*. New York: McCraw-Hill.

* If you see a patient looking distressed or clearly uncomfortable, stop!

* Similarly, if you are asked to do a procedure on a patient but feel really unsure about it, don't do it! Apply the Golden Rule– how would you like it if you were the patient? Would you allow the huge cut on you leg to be stitched by a trembling, clueless medical student who has never sutured a dummy? Express your concern to the doctor, even if this might be embarrassing. Temporary embarrassment is a far smaller price to pay than a permanent hideous scar caused by a medical student's poorly made sutures!

The moral obligations of medical students

Medical students, like everyone else, have to fulfil certain moral obligations. The article below, entitled *'how to be a good medical student'*, uses the ethical violations by medical students in Bristol as a springboard for discussion.

Article: How to be a good medical student

In early January 2003, a study led by Dr Coldicott appeared in the British Medical Journal revealing that nearly a quarter of rectal and vaginal examinations on anaesthetised patients were performed by medical students without patient consent.[4] Although the study did not generate the firestorm of controversy many expected, it engendered much discussion on ethical issues surrounding informed consent and patient autonomy, as well as stressing the need for greater ethics training for medical students. As an ethical problem, however, the case of intimate examinations is, to my mind, relatively uninteresting. If we agree that it is wrong for doctors to perform a vaginal examination on a *conscious* person without their consent, then it follows that it will still be wrong if that same person is merely asleep. Society would be somewhat chaotic if a person suddenly lost his rights when unconscious. The argument that the anaesthetised patient is unaware of the examination and so cannot be harmed is, at best, questionable. Suppose a newspaper revealed tomorrow that sociology students had placed hidden cameras in the cubicles of public toilets to study urination habits. Most people would be understandably outraged by this violation of privacy, even though the victims were not harmed by it at the time. This is based on the belief that a person's rights can be violated without that person's knowledge.

As for the conflict between the educational need of students and the respect for patient autonomy, it would only arise if an overwhelming number of patients refused to be examined. This is an unlikely scenario. In a commentary on Dr Coldicott's study, Britt-Ingjerd Nesheim, a professor of obstetrics and gynaecology in Norway, affirms that obtaining patient consent to student examinations is not difficult, as long as the patient feels comfortable with the arrangements.[5] Yet for me the study raises a more interesting question which extends beyond the recondite sphere of intimate examinations. It concerns the moral obligations of medical students faced with ethically dubious situations. In short, what should a 'good' medical student do?

In an article on the scope of medical ethics, Professor Raanan Gillon recounts two experiences from his days as a medical student.[6] The first describes his teacher's refusal to grant an abortion to a 14-year-old girl on the grounds that she was 'a slut'; the second his own refusal to examine a scrotal lump on a patient whose testicles had already been examined by five other students. Gillon's objections were very much the exception. When these events took place in the 1960s, medical students were simply expected to follow their teachers' orders and to absorb their evident wisdom without question. Since then, medical ethics has developed from an ill-defined embryonic subject to an academic discipline in its own right, with specific journals and associations, and a place in the medical curriculum.

Judging from some of the comments from students at Bristol, however, the growing emergence of medical ethics has not dispelled the awkward climate of unquestioned reverence towards teachers. Many of the students felt uneasy about the examinations, but were too intimidated to voice their concerns: "You couldn't refuse comfortably. It would be very awkward, and you'd be made to feel inadequate and stupid" commented a fourth year student who participated in the study. It seems clear that medical schools should strive to foster a climate more conducive to open discussion on ethical issues between students and teachers. Students should not have to perform heroic acts of courage to raise ethical concerns. In light of medical ethics' place in the curriculum, the situation is deeply paradoxical. Students may be taught the importance of respecting the patient's autonomy one day, but witness an obvious violation of this principle by their teachers the next. For the subject to be of any use, students must not only be allowed, but positively *encouraged* to put into practice their knowledge without the fear of appearing 'inadequate and stupid'. If a student's ethical concerns remain unresolved after discussion with the teacher, there should be formal methods of complaint, perhaps through a committee specifically set up for that purpose, or through the school's medical ethicist, who would then investigate the matter thoroughly. Medical ethics is, after all, an applied discipline.

It is nonetheless all too easy to blame the medical establishment and individual teachers for the unethical behaviour of students, as if the appellation 'medical student' shielded individuals from moral fault. In Nick Hornby's novel 'How to be good', the narrator, an adulterous GP and mother of two, resolves her moral conundrums by mechanically repeating 'I must be good. I'm a doctor'.[7] It is only later that she acknowledges that her justification is too facile: 'it's not enough to just be a doctor, you have to be a *good* doctor'. Students, however wide-eyed or intimidated, are still capable of independent thought. Their personal values should not vanish as they put on the white coat, just as a patient's rights should not evaporate when under anaesthetic. Although the reluctance of many Bristol students to perform the examinations is comforting, it seems that none acted on their qualms by declining to perform the procedure or asking that proper consent be obtained. Neither the diminished responsibility of the medical student, nor his status as an apprentice, removes the need for ethical reflection in daily proceedings. Indeed, far from absolving him from moral inquiry, these factors should encourage a process of ethical questioning. This exercise is, to my mind, crucial to a student's flourishing as a morally responsible future doctor. To modify Hornby's phrase 'it's not enough to just be a medical student'.

Notes:

- Ensure that a patient's consent is valid. Did the poor patient who 'consented' to have his testicles examined by five medical students really consent? Was he really free from undue influence at the time of the request?

- Even consultants make mistakes, and not just clinical ones! Don't do what your seniors tell you to if you strongly believe that they are wrong. Express your concerns.

- Use your nut.

> **A new form of advance directive?** Soon after writing the article above, I received an e-mail from a female reader, expressing disgust at the practice of intimate examinations without consent. She finished her e-mail: *I, meanwhile, am having my underwear embroidered with the words, "You do not have my consent for this"*.

Summary

- Respecting patient autonomy is, in normal circumstances, **ethically desirable** on consequentialist and deontological grounds.

- **Effective communication** is central to the process of obtaining informed consent.

- In some situations, when respecting patient autonomy would pose **considerable risks to others**, doctors should override the *prima facie* principle of respect for autonomy.

- Competent adults can refuse **any treatment**, including life-saving treatment.

- For incompetent adults, doctors should act in their **best interests**.

- What constitutes 'best interests' is not necessarily what is medically best, but depends on what is important to the particular patient.

- Taking **good medical notes** is crucial for the proper clinical management of the patient and for protecting you in case of legal action.

- Valid consent requires more than the signing of a consent form.

- Valid consent requires **freedom from pressure, good understanding and knowing enough** about the procedure to make an informed decision.

- Competence to consent is **specific** to a particular task.

- Patients must consent to involvement in medical teaching.

- Medical students, like doctors, have moral obligations to patients.

References

1. British Medical Association; Medical Ethics Today. London: BMJ Publishing Group, 2004:72.

2. General Medical Council. Seeking patient's consent: the ethical considerations.

3. Beauchamp T, Childress J. *Principles of Biomedical Ethics*. 5th ed. Oxford: Oxford University Press, 2001:72.

4. Coldicott Y, Pope C, Roberts C. The ethics of intimate examinations– teaching tomorrow's doctors. *British Medical Journal* 2003;326:97-99.

5. Nesheim B-I. Commentary: Respecting the patient's integrity is the key. *British Medical Journal* 2003;326:100.

6. Gillon R. What is medical ethics' business? *Advances in Bioethics* 1998;4:31-50.

7. Hornby N. *How to be good*. London: Penguin, 2001.

Secrets of a healthy relationship: the clinical relationship between doctor and patient

What is medical paternalism?

In medicine, paternalism refers to the **deliberate overriding or non-consultation of a patient's wishes with the intention of benefiting the patient or avoiding him harm.**

A useful distinction
Like tea, there are two types of paternalism: weak and strong

Weak paternalism: overriding or not consulting a patient's wishes in his best interests when the **patient is *inadequately* autonomous** (e.g. mad, delirious or very young).

Strong paternalism: overriding or not consulting a patient's wishes in his best interests when the **patient is *substantially* autonomous.**

Weak paternalism is not really controversial. It is obvious that others should make important decisions for people unable to make them. It would be irresponsible to let a delirious adult or a 5-year-old child decide whether to have life-saving surgery, for example. There is no real conflict between the principles of beneficence and respect for autonomy, since the patient has little autonomy to begin with.

Strong paternalism is much trickier, since the doctor overrides or does not consult a competent person's autonomous wishes. Strong paternalism has a bad reputation today, but throughout most of medicine's history, it was the dominant model of the doctor-patient relationship. Beneficence and non-maleficence triumphed over respect for autonomy. Since the 1960s, however, with the rise of individual rights, a shift has occurred and respect for autonomy is the strongest of the four principles in North America and the United Kingdom. Whether this should be so is the subject of much debate.

Arguments FOR paternalism:

- Doctors know more about medicine than patients, so they know what is best for them.

- The primary purpose of medicine is to make patients better and avoid harm (principles of beneficence and non-maleficence), so if this requires withholding some potentially harmful information or deceiving patients, then that is what doctors should do.

- Patients, in virtue of their illness and the unfamiliarity of their surroundings, are vulnerable and not at their best. They need doctors to make decisions for them.

Arguments AGAINST paternalism:

- Doctors may know what is in the *medical* best interests of their patients, but that's only one part of the concept of 'best interests'. Other things are important too, and only the individual patient can know what these are and how important they are to him. (see chapter 2)

- Strong paternalism often involves coercion, deception or withholding information, and therefore fails to respect patient autonomy. How can patients make adequately informed decisions if given false or incomplete information?

- Paternalism may cause more harm than good (for example, withholding information to avoid distress may prevent the patient from getting his affairs in order before his death). It may also be distressing to relatives and the medical team, who may well have to hide the truth from the patient.

- Some patients may be too sick to make autonomous decisions, but this doesn't mean that *all* patients will be incapable of autonomous choice. This is a logical fallacy.

Is strong paternalism ever justified?

By definition, strong paternalism violates patient autonomy. As we saw in the previous chapter, this is usually undesirable. Nevertheless, there may be rare cases where it is justified.

Beauchamp and Childress provide four conditions needed to justify strong paternalism (p. 186):[1]

1. The patient risks serious and preventable harm.

2. The paternalistic act will probably prevent the harm.

3. The likely benefits of the paternalistic act will outweigh the likely harms to the patient.

4. The alternative which least infringes patient autonomy is chosen.

> **An example of justified strong paternalism**
> John Smith, who is recovering from emergency thyroid gland surgery, is at risk of a lethal complication called 'thyrotoxic storm', which can be precipitated by stress. During post-operative tests, the doctor finds serious complications. Mr Smith asks a direct question about his health, which can only be truthfully answered by telling him about the complications. The doctor knows that revealing this information may cause the patient great distress. In this case, where respecting autonomy might lead to death or serious harm, deception may be the more humane option. Note, however, that the deception would only be temporary. Once the patient has recovered, the doctor would inform the patient of the complications.

Withholding information

Every doctor withholds information. No GP tells a patient with psoriasis about the location of the spleen, for example. A doctor has a duty, derived from the principle of respect for autonomy, to provide the patient with relevant information. Withholding relevant information can prevent patients from making reasoned and informed decisions.

Legally, the doctor should provide information **'in broad terms of the nature of the procedure which is intended'**.[2] This includes **diagnosis, prognosis, alternatives, likely side-effects and complications.**

To avoid negligence, two tests must be passed:

1. A doctor must act in accordance with a **responsible body of medical opinion** (i.e. the Bolam test).

2. The doctor should give warning of any significant risks which a **reasonable patient** would want to know.

A doctor cannot withhold information just because he thinks the patient will not consent if informed!

If the patient wants more information about the procedure, the doctor has a duty to provide the patient with this information in a clear and understandable manner.

There is no obligation, however, to inform patients of treatment options which the doctor considers futile.

Patients who don't want to know

If a patient tells you that he doesn't want to know everything, you should respect this, but **you must give him the basic facts of the procedure** otherwise the consent is not valid. You may want to gently encourage the patient to know a little more about his condition, if you think this is appropriate.

Truth-telling

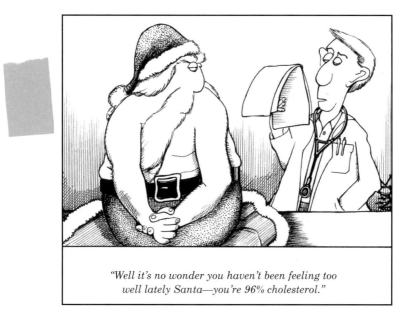

"Well it's no wonder you haven't been feeling too well lately Santa—you're 96% cholesterol."

Patients expect doctors to be honest and trustworthy. This expectation is central to the trust that exists between doctors and patients.

Why should doctors be truthful?

1. It respects patient autonomy and allows adequately informed consent.

2. It is the basis of trust between doctors and patients.

3. It coincides with our prima facie obligations of fidelity and promise-keeping.

> **Reminder:** a *prima facie* duty or obligation is one that must be respected unless it clashes with another *prima facie* duty, in which case balancing is needed to decide which duty should take priority.

Three common arguments FOR deception:

- Beneficence and nonmaleficence trump truth-telling. A doctor's **main priority is to improve patient health**. Telling the truth can harm the patient.

- The **truth can't be communicated** (i.e. the patient cannot possibly understand the truth, or the doctor is himself uncertain of the truth).

- **Patients don't want to know** the truth.

Arguments AGAINST deception:

- Deception **fails to respect autonomy**. Without the truth, patients may struggle to make informed decisions about the future.

- Patients are the **best judges of some of their interests**.

- Truthfulness **doesn't necessarily mean loss of hope**. The truth can be told in a way that maintains some hope. This is why doctors must have good communication skills. In the long term, it might be much better for the patient.

- Doctors risk hiding behind the principles of beneficence and nonmaleficence to avoid telling the truth. In other words, they can engage in **self-deception** to avoid the unpleasant task of disclosing bad news.

- Doctors must *try* to communicate what they think is true in accessible terms. If uncertain, they should **offer likelihoods** and share their uncertainty.

- Many people *would* want to be told the truth. Doctors often say that they would like to be told if in a similar situation! Besides, in an age of 'stranger' medicine (where patients are treated by a whole team of medics who do not know the patient very well), **patients often find out anyway!** At the outset, before any tests are performed, you could ask patients how much they would like to know. In many cases, they will want to be told everything. In some cases, however, they will leave the decision to inform at your discretion. Patients may have a **right to know** but they don't have **a duty to know** everything about their condition.

> *A cancer patient's perspective:*
> *"I would always wish to work with my doctor on terms of equal partnership. He brings his expertise, I bring my personal values and wishes. I would always want to be in control of my own destiny. In cancer, I would prefer quality of life to length of life i.e. I would not wish to have desperate measures in the form of chemotherapy in the end stages of the disease. Too many patients think that if chemo is offered this must mean that they can be 'cured'. Oncologists must learn to be totally honest: patients need to be able to make wills, see a grandchild, take a last holiday, and not spend their last months feeling sick and losing their hair and dignity."*

Situations when it is arguably OK to lie:

1. The lie is **trivial**, e.g. "I'm so sorry for getting you up in the middle of the night; I hope you don't mind, doctor, do you?".

2. **Emergencies**.

3. When telling the truth would cause **great and irreversible harm** (think of the patient at risk of thyrotoxic storm). Remember that telling the truth may cause short term harm (e.g. psychological harm) but may be desirable in the long term.

4. **Patient lacks competence** (for example, lying to a young child to give essential medication).

Article: Truth-telling and deception in medicine

The Italian poet Dante is not kind to deceivers. He condemns them to the very depths of hell, where they are whipped by horned demons and swim in the excrement they spouted to others whilst on earth. But do all deceivers deserve such punishment, in particular doctors who deceive patients with their best interests at heart? Are there instances when a doctor's deception is virtuous, rather than wicked? The use of deception in medicine is a sensitive subject. No one denies that it happens, but few are willing to tackle the issue full on.

Two years ago, an 18-year-old girl was admitted to a Canadian hospital, wishing to donate a kidney to her father. Despite six months on haemodialysis, her father's condition had declined rapidly and a kidney transplant was his last chance. Blood tests were requested to determine whether the two were compatible. When the results arrived, doctors discovered that the father and daughter were not biologically related, although they were compatible. The doctors were faced with an unsettling moral dilemma: should they tell their patients the truth or simply conceal the information?

In this instance, arguments can be found to support both disclosure and non-disclosure. On the one hand, informing the patients might destroy a close-knit family, dissuade the daughter from donating the life-saving kidney or even anger the patients who, after all, never asked to know this. On the other hand, doctors might invoke a duty to inform, or argue that the truth will out eventually and thus undermine the trust in the hospital and doctors generally. Finally, those in favour of disclosure could play one of the strongest cards in the medical ethics deck: the respect for patient autonomy. People are autonomous if they can make decisions based on their own beliefs, free from coercion and misleading information. In this case, the daughter is not making an autonomous decision as she clearly holds a *false* belief – that she is biologically related to her father. On this view, the doctors ought to correct the daughter's false belief by telling her the truth, thereby allowing her to make an informed decision.

In the end, the doctors agreed to inform the father and daughter of their unexpected finding. Although shaken by the revelation, the patients were glad that they were told, and the kidney transplant went ahead as planned.

The case just mentioned is rare, but situations involving deception are common in medical practice. There is a mismatch between the advice of the General Medical Council, which instructs doctors to be 'honest and trustworthy', and what goes on in the private consultation rooms of GPs and in hospital wards. At times, doctors do not tell elderly patients that they have terminal cancer. "The relatives beg us not to tell their darling mother that she has cancer, insisting that she'll just fall apart, and usually we comply" says a senior medical registrar who works in a major London hospital. Even in teaching hospitals, some doctors encourage students to use deception. In a recent issue of the student BMJ, a medical student wrote to the editor: 'for the second time our student group has been advised to lie when reporting patient information'. In January 2003, the BMJ revealed that a quarter of rectal and vaginal examinations on anaesthetised patients were performed by medical students without patient consent. When asked about the practice, a fourth-year medical student commented: "I was told in the second year that the best way to learn to do rectal examinations was when the patient was under anaesthetic. That way they would never know". Some doctors, to evade the awkward questions of patients, use carefully crafted language. One cancer specialist, when asked by a patient how long she had to live, replied "We deal with the living here". The patient interpreted this as several months, possibly years. A few days later, the patient met another doctor and asked him the same question. When the doctor informed her that she had only days to live, the patient was distraught. She died that same day. Last week, a medical student on a hospital placement told me that one of the surgeons introduces his students as 'junior doctors' to patients. Deceiving patients in this way erodes public trust in the medical profession, and undermines the laudable work of those other doctors who hold in higher esteem the relationship between doctors and patients. If the duty to tell the truth is not set in stone, it should at least be the default option.

Although in some cases deception is clearly wrong, there are times when it seems justified. The lies and deceptions of doctors need not lead to the lower circles of Dante's *Inferno*. What if a patient, the sole survivor of a fatal car crash, asks on her expiring breath about the fate of her young child who was also in the car? Should the doctor say that her daughter suffered gruesome injuries and died a slow death, or can he lie to reassure his dying patient? Here the desire to comfort a patient in her final moments arguably trumps the respect of a fleeting autonomy. What about lying to family members who enquire about the death of their loved one? "We often lie to relatives when the patient died horribly, especially if the relatives are clearly very distressed" comments the medical registrar. "Today, for example, a patient died really badly, vomiting litres of blood, and I told her relatives that she passed away peacefully in her sleep. I don't think it's wrong to lie in such cases". What about a patient with spinal injuries who, on the way to the operating theatre, asks the doctor whether he will ever walk again? Or the elderly patient, diagnosed with incurable metastatic cancer, about to go on a long-awaited holiday to Barbados? Can the doctor wait until the patient's return before breaking the bad news? Right or wrong, more research needs to be done on the use of deception in medicine, on its prevalence, its justifications, and in particular the beliefs of doctors, patients and members of the public on the matter. Only then can we aim to improve current practice and policy in ways that would be acceptable to all parties involved.[3]

Good communication skills

To respect patient autonomy, doctors should communicate information in a clear, comprehensible manner, and give patients opportunities to ask questions.

A good doctor should also communicate in a **compassionate and culturally-sensitive manner**. Remember the advice given in the previous chapter: 'use your nut!'. Try to imagine yourself in the patient's position. If delivering bad news, make sure you tell the truth without depriving the patient of all hope. **Do not just 'dump' the truth.** Ask questions to find out how much the patient wants to know. Different cultures have different norms regarding the disclosure of grim news. In Greece, Spain and Lebanon, for example, doctors tend to withhold diagnoses of cancer far more than in Britain and the United States. This does not mean that you should withhold such a diagnosis from a Spanish patient, of course, but you should **ask some exploratory questions** to discover how much that particular patient wants to know about his condition.

Good communication also helps to build a trustful relationship between doctor and patient. The BMA lists other advantages of effective communication (p. 34):[4]

1. Increases patient satisfaction and reduces the number of complaints.

2. Patients are more likely to adhere to their treatment.

3. Increases self care and self management activity.

4. Patients cope better with their condition.

5. Patients are less psychologically distressed and anxious.

What makes a good doctor?

In chapter 1, we introduced **virtue ethics**, which stresses the importance of the virtues in deciding right and wrong.

Now, it's obvious that being a good doctor requires more than technical competence. Many of the doctors struck off by the GMC are *technically* competent. They got past their Finals, after all! What some of them lack are certain character traits, such as honesty, compassion, responsibility and integrity.

The article below highlights the importance of reflection and certain character traits for the good practice of medicine. One of the ways to acquire the necessary virtues is by reading books. FHM or similar intellectual publications do not count.

Chapter 3

Article: Medicine, humanity and the humanities

'One of the hard things to learn in medicine' wrote Lewis Thomas 'is what it feels like to be a patient'. A hundred years ago, when serious illness was far more common than it is now, most doctors had themselves been very sick at one time or another. A doctor treating a patient with pneumonia may well have contracted the disease in the past. In consultations with his patient, the doctor would appreciate the hardships of living with the disease, having experienced them himself. Today, however, many doctors have never slept in a hospital bed or felt the fear and discomfort of serious illness. To remedy this lack of experience, Thomas suggested the invention of an 'illness simulator', akin to the sophisticated aircraft simulators used by trainee pilots. The 'illness simulator' would give medical students some idea of what it feels like to have pneumonia, cancer or multiple sclerosis. A single day of virtual pneumonia – chest pain, fever, coughing and all – might be enough to improve a doctor's bedside manner for life. Thomas made his suggestion with his tongue firmly embedded in his cheek, but the underlying point was serious: understanding what patients go through is essential to being a good doctor.

Short of an 'illness simulator', the most effective antidote to this common insensitivity is, quite simply, personal reflection. In a curriculum packed to the brim with ward rounds, lectures and practicals, medical students have little time to reflect on the nature of their chosen profession or, indeed, on the ultimate goals of medicine. 'Medical students have a very rigid timetable nowadays' commented a consultant endocrinologist working in London, 'when I trained as a doctor thirty years ago, we just followed doctors around!'. Any time outside the hospital is largely spent perusing medical textbooks in preparation for invariably frequent exams. It is unsurprising, then, that most medical students consider the study of medicine to be the memorisation of thousands of medical facts. The medical student has but one goal in mind: to pass finals and become a doctor; any work, any fact, that fails to contribute to this goal is deemed unimportant. It is a failure of our medical education that personal reflection, insight and understanding have been so evidently neglected in favour of factual knowledge. Even in a technological age, medicine is more than the mechanical application of medical facts to sick people. It is this excessive reliance on technology that largely explains why young doctors are ill-prepared to deal with the moral problems arising in medicine. In the last week of November 2003, the British Medical Association had 1400 visitors access its 'ethical advice' website. The following month, Michael Wilks, the chairman of the BMA ethics committee, announced in public that the many calls the BMA receives from distressed doctors indicate an urgent need to address moral issues at an early stage of medical training.

The chilling case of Dr Shipman has brought home the importance of moral character in the training and development of doctors. Technical competence without good character is more dangerous in medicine than in any other profession, partly because of the nature of a doctor's knowledge and partly because of the trust that patients have in their doctors. It is, after all, mainly because of his patients' trust that Shipman's crimes went undetected for so long. Although important, the careful selection of candidates at the admissions stage of medical school is not enough to ensure the combination of these two qualities. The teaching of moral reasoning and the encouragement of personal reflection must be an ongoing process throughout a doctor's career, from the first term at medical school onwards. Through regular meetings or seminars, medical students and doctors should be given opportunities to grapple with the feelings and moral problems that they encounter in the day-to-day life of the hospital.

History, philosophy and literature, by examining the nature of human experience through various lenses, provide insights into humanity that are highly relevant to the good and ethical practice of medicine. For these disciplines promote a greater understanding of medicine, its historical roots, its philosophical basis and its personal impact on both practitioners and patients. No medical textbook, for example, can convey the anxiety of a dying patient as well as a Tolstoy or a Solzhenitsyn. These texts are literary versions of the 'illness simulator'. Professor Jean Bernard, a renowned French haematologist, said in an interview "The doctor is a person always confronted with suffering and death. I have often found help and comfort in literature after a particularly hard day in the hospital".

Unlike in the United States, where students must go through years of general education before applying to medical school, most students in this country start studying medicine at eighteen and qualify as doctors at twenty-four. It is a young age at which to face death and suffering on a daily basis and to make important decisions affecting people's lives. A study published in 2000, which revealed that doctors are twice as likely to commit suicide than people in other professions, highlights the stress inherent in the job. The fostering of personal reflection, by examining the many facets of medical practice, will help young doctors practice their art with a clearer idea of the impact of illness on the lives of patients and their relatives, and a greater understanding of their profession. It may help them deal with the often harrowing experiences they encounter. When the poet Saint John Perse was asked why he wrote poems, he simply answered "to live better". If sceptics ask why medical students should study ethics and the humanities, a similar answer could be given: "to be better doctors".[5]

Summary

- There are two types of paternalism: **weak** and **strong**. Strong paternalism is the more controversial of the two.

- Strong paternalism may be justified in **very rare circumstances**.

- Being a good doctor requires more than mere technical ability or factual knowledge. Certain **virtues** are important.

- Doctors have a duty to provide **relevant information** to patients.

- If patients do not want to know the details of a procedure, doctors should provide only **basic facts** about the procedure.

- Doctors have a *prima facie* **duty of truth-telling** to their patients. This may be trumped by other duties in rare circumstances.

- Doctors should make sure they communicate information in a **clear and culturally-sensitive manner**, and **invite questions** from their patients.

References

1. Beauchamp T, Childress J. *Principles of Biomedical* Ethics. 5th ed. Oxford: Oxford University Press, 2001.

2. Chatterson v Gerson 1 QB 432, 1981.

3. Sokol D. Trust me, I'm a doctor. *The Independent* 2004;11.

4. British Medical Association; Medical Ethics Today. London: BMJ Publishing Group, 2004.

5. Sokol D. Take one Tolstoy with each meal. *The Times* 2004 13 March;7.

Keeping secrets: confidentiality and good clinical practice

What is medical confidentiality?

Confidentiality in medicine refers to **the protection of a patient's personal information from unauthorised parties** or, in simpler terms, keeping your patients' secrets!

Confidential information includes a patient's name and address, not just medical information.

Case example:
Feeling guilty, Adam Zapple calls the hospital to know whether the old granny he has just mugged (Ms Debbie Litate) is recovering well in hospital. The doctor tells Adam that Ms Litate is indeed a patient, but that her medical details cannot be disclosed on the grounds of respecting confidentiality.

Verdict: *By disclosing the patient's name, the doctor has breached patient confidentiality.*

Why is confidentiality important?

- To be a **good doctor** and **maintain the public trust** in the medical profession.

- To **avoid appearing in court** charged with breaking the law on confidentiality.

- To **avoid getting struck** off the register by the GMC. The GMC has erased several doctors for breaching confidentiality in previous years.

Confidentiality is a cornerstone of the doctor-patient relationship, mentioned clearly in the Hippocratic Oath. When patients consult doctors, they believe that the doctors will not disclose details of the consultation to third parties. Based on this belief, patients reveal even the most personal or embarrassing details to doctors safe in the knowledge that no one else will hear of them. Without a promise of confidentiality, however, **patients may be more reluctant to share information** with their doctor. They may decide not to visit the doctor at all. The doctors, lacking all the necessary information, will struggle to make an accurate diagnosis or suggest the most appropriate treatment. Confidentiality therefore **affects the therapeutic success of the consultation.**

If patients are aware that their electronic records are readily accessible by others, for example, they may withhold potentially vital information from their doctors or simply refuse to be hospitalised. One can easily imagine a patient with a sexually transmitted disease declining treatment for fear that relatives (who work at the hospital or know people who do) will discover a shameful 'secret' noted on the electronic record. So our resident consequentialist, Kevin, would most certainly stress the importance of confidentiality.

Confidentiality fosters trust between doctors and patients. Indeed, the word 'confidence' is composed of the Latin *con* ('with') and *fidere* ('to trust'). Doctors make an **implicit promise** to patients that information pertaining to their health will remain private. When we go to visit our GP, we assume that he will not discuss our large, ill-placed, pustulous growth to friends at a party. Violating confidentiality is violating the patient's *prima facie* right to privacy and **breaking the implicit promise between doctor and patient**. Repeated breaches of confidentiality will over time undermine the public trust in the medical profession. **Medical students, as part of the medical team, should abide by the same rules of confidentiality as doctors.**

Breaching confidentiality also fails to respect patient autonomy, since patients make decisions based on the belief that the doctor will not disclose personal information. Violating patient confidentiality is therefore a form of **betrayal**. After all, most of us feel betrayed when we discover that a friend has disclosed one of our secrets, even if they had good intentions. Dan the deontologist would consider respecting confidentiality as an important deontological rule.

Finally, Veronica the virtue ethicist might say that a **virtuous doctor,** who is honest, respectful, considerate, trustworthy and so on, would not reveal a patient's personal information to others without the patient's explicit permission or without an extremely good reason to do so.

> **Summary of reasons for maintaining patient confidentiality**
> 1. **Respecting the regulations of the GMC.**
>
> 2. **Respecting the legal duty of confidence.**
>
> 3. **Promise-keeping** (implicit promise that the doctor will not disclose personal information without the patient's permission).
>
> 4. **Consequentialism:** People will stop coming to the doctor or will not disclose everything in a consultation (loss of trust). This may lead to poor treatment and potential danger to others (think of an undiagnosed epileptic truck driver!).
>
> 5. **Respect for autonomy:** People rely on trust to arrange the nature of their relationship with others.
>
> 6. **Virtues:** Doctors should have virtues such as integrity, honesty, etc.

Confidentiality and children

- The confidentiality of children 16 or over should be respected. Therefore **the child's consent is required if the doctor wants to share information with the parents.**

- The confidentiality of children under 16 should be respected if they are deemed competent (i.e. Gillick competent). A child under 16 is Gillick competent if he has **'sufficient understanding and intelligence to enable him or her to *understand fully* what is proposed'.** (see chapter 8 for a brief account of the Gillick case)

- It is good practice to talk to the child about the possibility of informing the parents.

- As the patient is still a child, even if Gillick competent, the doctor should ultimately act in the child's best interests. Thus, there may be cases where a doctor believes disclosing the information to parents is in the child's best interests, even if the child protests. The doctor must have a good reason for acting in this way, however, and should be prepared to justify his decision.

• If the child is incompetent, doctors should generally disclose medical information to the parents.

When can doctors breach confidentiality?

Respecting patient confidentiality is a form of respecting patient autonomy, but remember that respect for autonomy can sometimes be overridden in certain circumstances, such as when it infringes the autonomy of others or in emergencies. Some of the legally required breaches of confidentiality stem from the belief that **doctors have duties to society that override their duties to individual patients.**

If you do have to disclose information, make sure you **disclose the minimum necessary for the purposes.** For example, if the Chief Officer of Police asks you for details of a driver who ran over a pedestrian (invoking the Road Traffic Act 1988), you should give the name and address of the patient, *not* details of his medical history unless the patient consents to this or a court of law demands it.

When are doctors legally required to breach confidentiality?

• **Notifiable disease** – If the patient has a notifiable disease (such as tuberculosis, meningitis, typhoid fever, viral haemorrhagic fevers, plague or food poisoning), doctors are required **by law** to get in touch with the 'proper officer' of their local authority. It is good practice to explain to the patient why this is necessary. Some of the notifiable diseases, notably the viral haemorrhagic fevers, are easily transmittable diseases which could cause thousands of fatalities in short time periods. Failing to notify the appropriate authorities about such diseases can have disastrous consequences for others.

Did you know?
In the Middle Ages, doctors commonly abandoned their patients during severe and widespread epidemics. When the plague reached Venice, for example, doctors fled in flocks to avoid contagion. The problem got so bad that many European cities passed laws forbidding doctors to run away during epidemics!

Chapter 4

- **Court order** – If a court orders you, either orally in court or in writing, to hand over some confidential information, you are legally required to do so. Failure to do can lead to imprisonment! If you are not in court, make sure you actually see the written order. Don't rely on other people's word! ("Hi Dr Jones, I'm, uh, Mr Smith's lawyer, please send me your patient's medical record, I've got a court order!")

- **Births and abortions** – Doctors or midwives should notify the district medical officer of births within 6 hours.

  For abortions, the doctor should inform the Chief Medical Officer of the abortion, and provide the name and address of the woman (Abortion Act 1967).

- **Infertility** – All people undergoing infertility treatment and all children born from the treatment must be registered with the Human Fertilisation and Embryology Authority (HFEA). The doctor should therefore give the names of these people (i.e. the people undergoing treatment and any resulting babies) to the HFEA so they can put the details on their register.

- **Road Traffic Act (1998)** – If the Chief Officer of Police asks a doctor for details of a person suspected of a driving offence, the doctor should provide them with the name and address of the patient. Note that this doesn't just apply to doctors, but to everyone.

- **Terrorism** – It is a criminal offence not to inform a police constable of a belief or suspicion of terrorist activity 'as soon as is reasonably practicable' (Terrorism Act 2000, chapter 11). Nevertheless, a later Act added that you are off the hook as long as you have a 'reasonable excuse for not disclosing the information' (Anti-terrorism, Crime and Security Act 2001, chapter 24).

When do doctors have discretion on whether to breach confidentiality?

Some situations are left to the discretion of clinicians. The GMC describes some of these circumstances.

> **From the GMC booklet** *Serious Communicable Diseases* **(1997)**
> 'You may disclose information about a patient, whether living or dead, in order to protect a person from risk of death or serious harm. For example, you may disclose information to a known sexual contact of a patient with HIV where you have reason to think that the patient has not informed that person, and cannot be persuaded to do so. In such circumstances you should tell the patient before you make the disclosure, and you must be prepared to justify a decision to disclose information.'[1]
>
> Note that you should not tell any others who are *not* at serious risk of harm.

- **HIV and AIDS** – If a patient is HIV positive, the doctor should discuss with the patient ways to minimize the risk of infecting others, especially sexual partners. If the patient refuses to change his behaviour or to tell sexual partners about his condition, **the patient's confidentiality may be breached to protect others from serious risk.**

- **Public safety** – Think of an epileptic taxi driver who refuses to stop driving, or of an alcoholic plane pilot! If, after several attempts to explain the situation to a patient who you think might endanger others, the patient still refuses to do anything about it, you may want to alert the police. In the case of potentially dangerous drivers, you can alert the Driver and Vehicle Licensing Agency (details in appendix D). In these situations, you should balance the harms and benefits of disclosing the information. You should consider, for example, the **likelihood** of the harm occurring and the gravity of the harm if it does occur.

- **Serious crime** – Think of a modern-day Jack the Ripper entering your surgery. If you reasonably suspect that one of your patients has committed, or is about to commit, a serious crime (e.g. murder, rape, kidnapping) you should contact an appropriate person or authority. (Note: if the patient is a terrorist, you are legally required to inform the police!). So, unless your patient is a known terrorist, you should balance the harms and benefits of disclosing the information, and you should disclose no more than what is absolutely necessary. Some crimes are worse than others, of course. Stealing an apple is quite different in seriousness to blowing up a government building. It is unlikely that breaching confidentiality to report the theft of an apple will protect public safety.

- **Risk of harm to patients or others** – If maintaining your patient's confidentiality poses a risk of death or serious harm to the patient or others, you are justified in disclosing the information to a relevant authority without your patient's consent. This includes child abuse (see below).

- **Domestic violence and abuse of children**

Below is the advice of the GMC on this:

'If you believe a patient to be a victim of **neglect or physical, sexual or emotional abuse** and that the patient **cannot give or withhold consent to disclosure,** you should give information **promptly** to an **appropriate responsible person or statutory agency,** where you believe that the disclosure is in the patient's best interests. You should **usually inform the patient** that you intend to disclose the information before doing so. Such circumstances may arise in relation to children, where concerns about possible abuse need to be shared with other agencies such as social services. Where appropriate you should inform those with parental responsibility about the disclosure. If, for any reason, you believe that disclosure of information is not in the best interests of an abused or neglected patient, you must still be prepared to justify your decision.' (GMC, *Confidentiality: protecting and providing information*)[2]

Special cases and important points

- Confidential information may be disclosed to others with the patient's consent.

- Don't breach patient confidentiality for trivial reasons or to amuse your friends in the pub, however tempting this may be. An overdose of wine gums is *not* a valid excuse for disclosure.

- Your duties are **to your patient** first and foremost. Ask the patient for permission first, even if relatives want to know. Relatives have no legal status in law.

What to avoid – a true example of unethical behaviour:
From a PRHO: "My senior doctor always tells the relatives first if he discovers a patient has terminal cancer. He'll only tell the patient if the relatives say that's fine. A lot of the time, the relatives ask him not to say anything, so the patient never knows!"

- Once data is anonymised and the patient cannot be identified, the information is no longer confidential. Nevertheless, it is courteous and good practice to obtain the patient's permission.

- Whether or not a patient can be identified depends in part on the rarity of the condition. So, although there would be little chance of identifying a patient with halitosis from London, it would be much easier to identify a patient with Gorham's disease (an *extremely* rare bone disorder) living in Wells, Somerset, allegedly England's smallest city.

- The GMC, as well as many medical journals, advise doctors who publish patients' case histories or photographs in a journal to obtain patient consent, even if they cannot be recognised.

- Tell patients if their personal information will be shared with other members of the healthcare team, and explain to them why this is important. If they refuse, you should respect this, unless there is a risk of serious harm to others. Note that this does not apply in an emergency.

- Even after a patient's death, confidentiality should generally be respected, although you may have to provide information to the coroner (whose duty is to investigate violent, sudden or unnatural deaths) or Procurator Fiscal, on death certificates, or as part of national enquiries. If relatives ask for information about the patient's illness, the BMA suggests that you should 'weigh the benefits to the patient's partner or family of disclosing information against the duty of confidentiality.'(p. 179)[3] In practice, this means that, unless the patient told you to keep the medical details a secret, it is probably acceptable to share them with the relatives. Needless to say, compassion is key when sharing such delicate information.

- If the police request confidential information about a **serious** crime, breaching patient confidentiality may be justified. Nevertheless, ask the police to justify the request in writing. If working in A&E, take down the police officer's name, phone the police station and ask for the person. This provides a pretty good guarantee that the caller is in fact a police officer!

In practice – avoiding unintentional breaches of confidentiality

It is surprisingly easy to breach confidentiality by accident. The Medical Protection Society (MPS) have provided a list of common situations where such breaches occur.

- **Lifts and canteens.** It is always risky to discuss patients in a public place, but in small, crowded places, it becomes high risk! You can easily mention identifying information within earshot of others. You need to be cautious, even if you think the only people around are healthcare professionals.

- **A&E departments and wards.** Again, these are places where patients, relatives and friends are in close proximity to doctors. If you need to talk to a colleague about a patient, make sure you cannot be overheard.

- **Computers, faxes and printers.** It is common, particularly in general practice, for patients to openly see computer screens showing confidential patient information. This is clearly unacceptable.

Occasionally, doctors update a patient's notes on the computer in the consulting room and leave the details on the screen when the next patient comes in. The notes of patients should not be visible to other patients.

When sending sensitive information to a fax or printer make sure the receiving machine is in a secure place where only authorised people can access it.

- **Patient notes.** Patient records are confidential documents. Be careful about who can see them. Never leave notes in an area with open access. Only allow people to see the notes if they need them for their job. Many doctors have faced complaints by patients who saw the confidential notes of other patients stacked on the receptionist's desk.

Confidentiality is central to a healthy doctor-patient relationship. On both consequentialist and deontological grounds, respecting patient confidentiality is desirable. **It ensures that patients feel free to disclose even the most embarrassing information, it helps doctors make accurate diagnoses and prescribe the right treatments, it fosters trust in the medical profession, and it respects patient autonomy.** Nevertheless, it is not an absolute obligation. There are cases where the doctor should consider breaching confidentiality, such as when the patient might cause serious harm to others. The decision must take into account the harms and benefits of violating this important principle. At times, the doctor is **legally required** to disclose confidential information, such as when the patient is infected with a notifiable disease. In each case, doctors should be able to **justify their decision** by appealing to both ethical principles and the law. The justifications will invariably involve an elaboration and weighing of the Four Principles of medical ethics: respect for autonomy, beneficence, non-maleficence and justice.

Summary

* Confidentiality is a **legal** and **ethical requirement** in the doctor-patient relationship.

* Confidentiality may be breached if the patient consents to sharing the information, or in certain cases where breaching confidentiality is in the public interest (e.g. if respecting confidentiality poses a threat of serious harm to others or in cases of suspected child abuse).

* The confidentiality of children over 16 should be respected.

* For 'Gillick competent' children under 16, confidentiality should also be respected unless the doctor deems that this is not in the best interests of the child.

* Doctors should ensure that patient confidentiality is not breached **unintentionally** (e.g. in lifts, canteen, A&E department).

* Doctors should be able to **justify their decisions** to respect or breach patient confidentiality.

References

1. General Medical Council. Serious Communicable Diseases.

2. General Medical Council. Confidentiality: protecting and providing information.

3. British Medical Association; Medical Ethics Today. London: BMJ Publishing Group, 2004.

Lab rats and human guinea pigs: research, innovative treatment and clinical audit

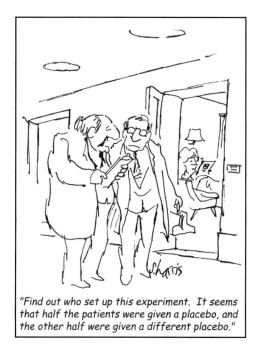

"Find out who set up this experiment. It seems that half the patients were given a placebo, and the other half were given a different placebo."

Why do research?

Why is it a good thing for doctors to conduct medical research? Why do we bother at all? The answer lies in the **principle of beneficence:** we have a duty to do good for our patients. To achieve this, we must know which treatments work and which don't. We should also strive to improve existing treatments or, in cases where none exist, to discover new ones. This cannot be done without medical research.

Although medical research harbours great hopes, from healing the blind to providing a cure for cancer, the phrase 'medical research' conceals a darker side. The history of medical research is strewn with abuses. Some of the most infamous examples of unethical research were carried out in the 1940s by Nazi doctors (see box overleaf).

> **'Medical Research' in Nazi Germany**[1]
> **Antibiotic testing:** Nazi doctors inflicted wounds on prisoners of war. To simulate realistic battlefield wounds, doctors tied off blood vessels to interrupt the blood supply to the wound. The wounds were then deliberately infected with bacteria, such as *Clostridium perfringens* (which causes gas gangrene) and *Clostridium Tetani* (which causes tetanus). Wood shavings and ground glass were forced into the wounds to aggravate infection. The purpose of the study was to test the effectiveness of new antibiotics such as Sulfanilamide against wound infections. Many subjects died from the injuries.
>
> **Sea water experiments:** Various chemical methods to make sea water drinkable were trialled on prisoners of war. Subjects were deprived of all food and given only chemically processed sea water to drink. The results were often fatal.
>
> **Vaccine and drug trials:** Doctors deliberately infected thousands of subjects with virulent pathogens such as malaria, typhus, cholera and diphtheria to test vaccines and drugs against these infections. Several hundred prisoners died or suffered serious permanent disabilities.

Who regulates medical research?

Medical research is guided heavily by the ethical principles set out in the **Declaration of Helsinki**.[2] This document was drafted by the World Health Organisation in 1964 as a result of international pressure following the wartime atrocities. It remains the foundation for all other guidance on medical research.

In the past, research was largely self-regulated, but this is no longer the case. In 2001, the Department of Health's *Research governance framework for health and social care* recommended that all research be independently reviewed to ensure that it meets ethical standards.[3] Review by an **Ethics Committee** is now a **legal requirement,** under the Clinical Trials Regulations (2004) which implemented the European Clinical Trials Directive (Directive 2001/20/EC) in UK law.

Ethics committees are made up of doctors, nurses, other professionals (e.g. ethicists, lawyers, theologians), and lay persons.

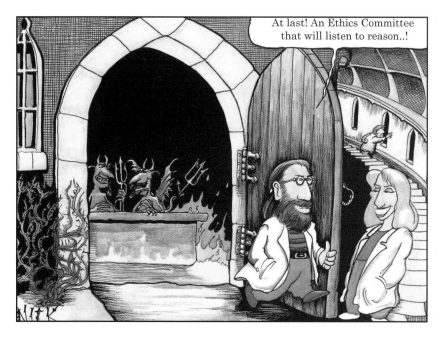

What explains this shift toward increased regulation? Firstly, ethically dubious research did not end with the Declaration of Helsinki in the 1960s. Researchers have conducted questionable medical research in the very recent past and, no doubt, some continue to do so today! The **public climate** in which research is carried out also has an impact. The recent public outcry over organ retention at a number of hospitals (see box below) illustrates the need to make research procedures transparent and acceptable to the public.

Organ retention at Alder Hey

In 1998, Britain witnessed a media outcry over the covert retention of organs at Alder Hey Children's Hospital in Liverpool. Similar organ collections were later revealed in Bristol and Birmingham. In fact, the practice was widespread: a 1999 census found that 210 NHS trusts and medical schools were holding over 100,000 organs, body parts, and entire corpses of stillborn babies and fetuses.

Few doubt that the organs were retained with good intentions. Pathologists can gather valuable information on the causes of death in children from such material. Yet many families were greatly distressed by the revelations.

Some commentators argued at the time that consent had been given since parents had signed the post-mortem form. This form included a clause consenting to the **retention of tissue samples**. Whether organs might be called 'tissue samples' is controversial. Even if we accept this interpretation, it is clear that the parents did not understand that organs could be removed when they signed the form. *Valid consent was therefore not obtained.*

Commenting on the case, the Royal College of Pathologists stressed the importance of explaining to families the exact nature of what was being proposed. Any paternalistic notions that the 'full details might be too distressing to families' were rejected. Many families now say that they might have been willing to donate organs for research had they been asked.

Types of medical research

The term 'medical research' covers a wide range of activities, from cells in the test tube to studies involving human subjects. For medical students, the main areas to be aware of are:

• Research (used in the strict sense of the word)

• Innovative treatment

• Clinical audit

The differences between these are summarized below:

RESEARCH:
• Aims to produce **new knowledge** that can be generally applied in the future, using rigorous scientific methods.

• Is NOT intended to benefit participants **directly** (although incidental benefit may occur).

• Will benefit **future generations** of patients.

INNOVATIVE TREATMENT:
- Aims both to **advance knowledge** and to benefit the **participant**.

- The *primary* consideration is to achieve the best outcome for **that patient**, regardless of knowledge gained along the way.

- May be conducted on a **one-off** or **small numbers basis**, outside the context of a properly described protocol.

CLINICAL AUDIT:
- Clinical audit is a process that **compares** the care actually received by patients with current 'best practice' standards.

- Ensures that the current knowledge base is **used optimally**, rather than adding to it.

Ethical issues in research and innovative treatment

1. Respect for autonomy: informed consent, truth-telling and adequate provision of information.
Patients should *always* be told if they are going to be involved in research. The only exceptions might be when a patient's mental capacity is impaired, or in the areas of research into emergency treatment, resuscitation and intensive care.

Obtaining adequately informed consent is just as important for medical research as for any other clinical situation. Indeed, it may be even **more important** to give patients adequate and honest information in the research setting since the potential risks and benefits are less certain.

In the past, some patients have been included in research **without** their consent. One justification for this was that informing patients of the situation would influence the outcome of the study. However, such a policy is no longer permitted.

The case of Mrs Thomas[4]

Mrs Thomas had a mastectomy for breast cancer in the early 1980s. While recovering from the operation, she realised that the patient in the neighbouring bed was receiving significantly different care. Unlike Mrs Thomas, the other patient had received postoperative counselling from a specialist nurse. The discrepancy was not explained to Mrs Thomas.

Four years later she discovered that she had been included in a trial to evaluate the effects of counselling versus no support following mastectomy. These trials were carried out over 5 years at 58 centres, and involved over 2000 women *without their consent*.

The health professionals involved in the research chose not to inform patients, on the grounds that they [the health professionals] would find it too upsetting to explain the situation. The Research Ethics Committee allowed them to proceed without the normal consent procedure.

Mrs Thomas complained to the Health Service Commissioner. The Committee on the Parliamentary Commission for Administration expressed considerable concern about the conduct of the study.

Such cases can result in a number of undesirable consequences:

- Patients might feel **hurt and angry** if they discover that they have been deceived or unwittingly 'used' as part of a study.

- Patients might **lose trust** in their doctors and may decide not to seek treatment in the future.

- There may be a **loss of public confidence** in research and the medical profession in general.

Doctors should **always** obtain adequately informed consent from patients before involving them in any form of medical research.

2. Beneficence and Non-maleficence

As we explained earlier, the principle of beneficence includes a duty to support medical research. However, the research must be conducted within a morally acceptable framework. A key principle in research ethics is **non-maleficence**. We have a strong duty not to harm those who help us acquire new medical knowledge.

Although there is a degree of risk inherent in any medical intervention, the issue of risk is particular important in medical research, as participants do not usually benefit from the research. Researchers have a duty to **minimize all foreseeable risks,** even with the valid consent of participants. Some consequentialists would take issue with this, and argue that significant expected gains might justify exposing participants to greater degrees of risk.

Point of debate in research ethics : what constitutes 'minimal' risk?

The Declaration of Helsinki states that research subjects should be exposed to 'minimal risks' only. But how much risk is 'minimal'? And how much risk should we allow consenting adults to take?

Some feel it is *unreasonably paternalistic* to prevent people from taking higher risks if they freely consent to do so. This is known as the **Libertarian position**. Libertarians point out that people are allowed to take significant risks in other areas of life. We are all free to go bungee jumping, bull-fighting, or to cycle on a main road without a helmet.

How can 'risk' be meaningfully assessed?

Curiously, angling is recorded as the UK's most dangerous sport, as it kills more people each year than any other (usually by drowning!). Yet few would use this as a reason to ban angling. The case of angling illustrates the difficulty of trying to accurately reflect the level of risk involved in some activities. Assessing risk can be complicated. It is not enough to look only at the number of injuries resulting from an activity. A quick look at accident statistics reveals that few everyday activities are totally safe:

- Over 10,000 Britons are hurt annually in accidents involving **socks and tights**.

- Last year, incidents involving **bird baths** accounted for 311 trips to casualty.

- 3421 people are injured by their **clothes baskets** each year.[5]

If we considered the level of risk involved in walking to the corner shop to buy milk, we might never leave the front door. So how can we convey the level of risk involved in research to potential participants?

> For the Royal College of Physicians (1996), 'minimal risk' represents (p. 197):[6]
>
> - a common event where the **level of distress is slight**, such as a mild headache, or
>
> - one where the **chance of serious injury** is very remote.
>
> Compared to the everyday risks we take, 'minimal risk' might be comparable to travelling on public transport or in a private car but *not* travelling by bike or motorcycle.

As previously mentioned, a number of ethicists favour the **Libertarian position.** They argue that people should be allowed to take greater risks while participating in research, as long as they *freely consent* to it. After all, they can refuse life-saving treatment at risk of certain death!

What might be wrong with this position?

> **Lawrence the Libertarian** has an exciting idea for a research project. Based on his vast personal experience, he has come up with the hypothesis that *one-eyed medical students do better in exams than students with a complete visual apparatus.*
>
> He reasons that one-eyed students are less distracted in the library, as their peripheral vision is poorer. They therefore spend more time reading and revising than ogling lycra-clad rowers.
>
> He proposes to remove one eye from a group of his medical student colleagues, and to compare the exam performance of his cycloptic subjects with that of their two-eyed rivals. Lawrence recruits 10 willing volunteers at the annual medical school beer-fest and puts his research proposal before the Local Research Ethics Committee.
>
> Unfortunately for Lawrence, the Committee rule that the removal of an eye is an unacceptable risk to allow the students to take, even if they are willing and the potential knowledge gained from the study might be valuable.

Although my research idea was ... sorry, Lawrence's idea was undoubtedly an extreme one, there may well be good reasons to **limit** the sorts of risks we allow people to take for research. These include the obligation to **avoid causing net harm,** the need to **maintain public trust** in the medical profession, and the **desire to avoid litigation.**

3. Justice

We have considered the possible harms of taking part in medical research, but what about the harms of being excluded from research? Conducting research on certain groups raises additional ethical issues. Consider the case of patients severely disabled by stroke. As they are unable to consent for themselves, the simple solution would be to exclude them from research studies. However, this might result in a complete lack of new treatments for this disabling condition.

If we routinely exclude certain groups from research studies, we will end up with **no proven treatments** for these groups. It is therefore important to include a **wide range** of patients in medical research, including members of ethnic minority groups, children and incapacitated adults. The difficulty lies in finding ethically acceptable ways to do this.

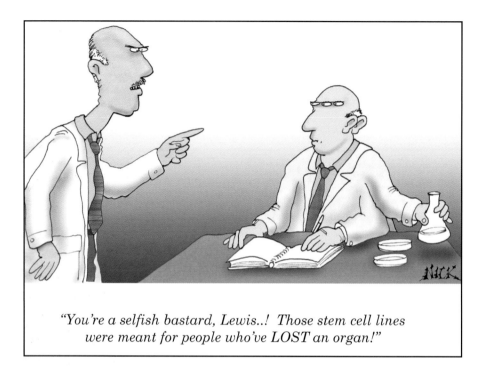

"You're a selfish bastard, Lewis..! Those stem cell lines were meant for people who've LOST an organ!"

Special considerations for vulnerable groups

People unable to consent

Research should only be conducted on incompetent patients if:

- The research cannot be carried out on consenting adults instead.

- It is likely to benefit either the incompetent patient himself or patients suffering from the same condition as the patient.

The capacity to consent may vary widely within such groups and should be carefully assessed on an individual basis. It is also good practice to **involve the families** of adults unable to consent in the decision. In Scotland, proxy decision makers can act for the incapacitated adult in certain circumstances. In England, however, there is no proxy consent for adults.

Children

We also need to carry out research on children, as they have a different physiology to adults and suffer from specific illnesses that do not affect adults. The decision to take part in research rests with the **child himself if he is competent** (see chapter 8) and **his parents if he is not**. Even if the child is competent, it is still good practice to obtain parental consent.

In addition, if the child clearly **objects** to a non-therapeutic procedure carried out for research purposes, doctors should **not proceed**, even with parental consent.[7] Children can become distressed by relatively minor procedures, such as having blood taken. If these procedures are not essential for their clinical care it is wrong to subject children to them whatever the expected gains for the research itself.

Healthy Volunteers

Healthy volunteers are an invaluable part of many research projects. However, the source and payment of these volunteers has often been criticized. Traditionally, researchers have called upon students, colleagues and lab workers to participate in their research. This raises concerns about the **voluntariness** of their decision to participate. For example, a PhD student may feel compelled to participate in his supervisor's research project for fear of damaging their relationship. The GMC now emphasizes that the recruitment of people in a 'dependent relationship', such as students or junior staff from the researcher's department, should be avoided.[8]

> **Fun fact:** For centuries, researchers have experimented on themselves. In 1984, Barry Marshall, an Australian gastroenterologist, demonstrated that *Helicobacter pylori* caused peptic ulcers by downing a flask of water full of the bacteria. Following an unpleasant bout of nausea and vomiting, a gastric biopsy revealed acute gastritis and the presence of H. Pylori bacteria. We do not recommend trying this at home!

Give me the money!

What about the issue of payment? Financial incentives are commonly used to attract volunteers. While paying people to take part in research is not in itself unethical, there are several conditions to fulfil:[7]

- Payment must **not be paid for undergoing risk**.

- The financial incentives should not act as an '**inducement**' to participate against the better judgment of the subject, nor to take part '**more frequently than is advisable**' (exactly how frequently is 'not advisable' is not specified).

- The issue of payment should be **monitored** by Research Ethics Committees.

Despite the conditions, we all know that most medical students volunteer for research trials for the money! How realistic these conditions are is therefore open to question.

Therapeutic versus non-therapeutic research – an outdated concept?

Since the 1960s, research on human subjects has been traditionally divided into two categories:

1. **Therapeutic** (or 'clinical') **research** – aimed to **improve patient care**, akin to what we now call 'innovative treatment'.

2. **Non-therapeutic research** – aimed to **produce new knowledge**, without benefiting participants.

Historically, the Declaration of Helsinki saw a fundamental distinction between the two types of research. Therapeutic research was less tightly regulated than non-therapeutic research. This was to allow easy access to experimental treatments for patients with no existing therapy options. Today, the World Health Association sees this distinction as **outdated and unhelpful**, as some forms of therapeutic research might be equally or more dangerous than non-therapeutic research. Furthermore, many procedures in therapeutic research may, in themselves, be non-therapeutic. This raises a number of questions: are these non-therapeutic procedures necessary? Does the patient know that they are non-therapeutic? Can the patient distinguish between what constitutes part of his treatment and what is additional for the purposes of experiment or monitoring?

In fact, one could argue that we need extra safeguards where research is combined with the treatment of sick people. In the absence of other treatment options, desperately ill and vulnerable patients might agree to risky experimental treatments against their better judgement. However, there is **some distinction** between research and innovative treatment relating to the conditions that studies must fulfil.

What do we need to tell patients about research projects?

For **research projects** where the aim is to gain new knowledge (rather than solely to care for the patient), **patients should be told:**

- The clear **purpose** of the research.

- Whether they are **likely to benefit** from the research.

- The **likely risks** and **benefits** (if they stand to benefit).

- The **difference** between medical research and ordinary treatment.

- **What is involved in the study,** including meanings of terms such as *randomisation.*

- **Alternative treatments** outside the study (if applicable).

- That they can **refuse or withdraw** at any time.

- That **refusal to participate** in research **will not affect the care** they receive.

- Details of **compensation** if they are harmed.

- Any **vested interests** of the researcher.

In the case of **innovative treatment**, the conditions differ slightly from those of pure research. **Patients must be told:**

- **How and why** the proposed innovative treatment **differs** from standard therapy.

- What **alternative treatments** (including standard therapies) are available.

- The **evidence** for the innovative treatment and any **uncertainties** about it. In controlled trials, patients should also be told the **evidence for the alternatives.**

- **How much experience** the doctor treating them has in the proposed technique.

- The **support available** if something goes wrong.

- The **likely future use** of the therapy if successful.

You will notice that the requirements for information giving in research and innovative treatment are much **more stringent** than in ordinary patient care. Some authors argue that this amounts to double standards between research and everyday care.[6] Can these apparent double standards be justified? Several reasons can be given to justify the difference:

- The **level of uncertainty is usually higher** in experimental treatments than in established treatments.

- Patients often hold a '**therapeutic misconception**'. In brief, they assume that a) what is new is necessarily an improvement (although it may turn out to be worse than the standard care) and b) that whatever is done to them is always for their benefit, even if told otherwise!

- In everyday practice there is no need to tell patients about areas of uncertainty, as we select the optimum treatment for the patient based on clinical experience.

- Routinely giving patients all this information in the clinical setting would take up huge amounts of time. Spending so long on explanation might actually be detrimental to patient care – there would be little time to do any work!

Whatever their views on the arguments above, doctors need to provide patients with **additional information** when offering them innovative therapies.

Requirements for clinical audit

The medical team caring for a patient does **not need to obtain consent** to use his records for audit, nor does this activity have to be overseen by an ethics committee. The consent of patients to use records for audit is believed to be *implied,* as long as patients are **generally aware that audit exists.**[7]

Sometimes audit is carried out by people outside the clinical team. If data are anonymised, no consent is needed. However, researchers often want to review non-anonymised records. If possible, they should obtain the consent of patients, but this may be unrealistic if large numbers of records are needed. Some patients might feel uneasy about the use of their health records for this purpose. Still, the Health and Social Care Act 2001 may allow such use if the research is clearly in the *wider public interest.*

A note on Randomised Controlled Trials

Randomised Controlled Trials (RCTs) are increasingly used in clinical research, as they are the most scientifically robust way to compare treatments. However, we should only use RCTs where there is *no recognised optimum treatment* for a condition, or where a new treatment is thought to be *significantly better* than existing therapies.

Involving a patient in a RCT is only ethical when there is **substantial uncertainty** about the best way to treat that particular patient, regardless of any general questions we may want the trial to answer. Some patients find the uncertainty of not knowing which treatment they will receive uncomfortable. Patients who have any preferences about their treatment should not be included in RCTs. Researchers should always discuss with patients all treatment options outside the RCT to establish if they have any preferences.

Good and bad research

It is vital to ensure that research is of **good quality**, both to justify the risks to the participants and to ensure that future patients are not harmed by misleading conclusions. To be of 'good quality', research must address **clearly defined questions** using **systematic and rigorous methods**. Research projects must meet certain minimum standards:

Minimum standards for research projects:[7]

- Well conducted project.

- Statistically significant numbers of subjects.

- Not an unnecessary duplication of previous research (i.e. do a good literature search before you begin!).

- External review and continuing surveillance.

- Special considerations for dependent or vulnerable subjects.

Fraud and misconduct in medical research

In the past, the names of senior researchers were often added to research papers, even if they had contributed nothing. This was known as 'gift authorship'. Although still common, it is now regarded as a highly dubious practice.

True story: fraudulent research and public disgrace⁹

In 1996, an obstetrician published a paper reporting the birth of a baby following the re-implantation of an ectopic pregnancy. This 'medical breakthrough' generated a certain amount of media interest. The name of the President of the Royal College of Obstetricians and Gynaecologists was included on the paper as a 'gift author'.

The first author also published a randomised controlled trial at the same time. **Both papers were later exposed as fraudulent.** Neither the patient seemingly involved in the first paper, nor those in the RCT could be traced. This was because *the patients did not exist*. An investigation into this doctor's work revealed three more fraudulent research papers, dating back to 1989. The doctor lost his job and was struck off by the GMC.

The president of the Royal College had to resign from all his positions, even though he was unaware that the work was fraudulent.

It was also common not to disclose conflicts of interest in research. Today, this omission is regarded as serious misconduct. The results of medical research can have immediate implications for people – just think of the Lancet paper which showed a link between the MMR vaccine and autism.[10] Take-up rates for the vaccine fell dramatically from over 90% to under 80%.[11] Bad research can also affect the **public perception** of doctors and researchers, undermining public trust in the scientific community. For these reasons, scientists have a moral obligation to conduct research in good faith, avoiding conflicts of interests and the pitfalls of bias.

Research on animals

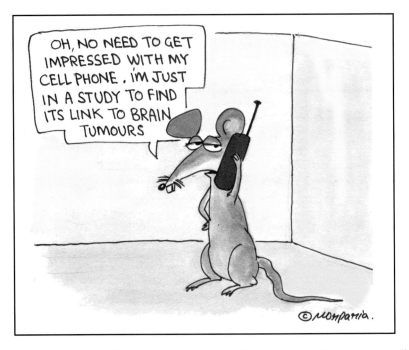

Experiments on animals have been a major contributor to **many important medical advances** in the recent history of medicine. This includes the development of vaccines, antibiotics, kidney transplants and open heart surgery. Experiments on animals are still of great relevance today, especially with the advent of transgenic animals. Many medical students will have participated in animal research during the course of their studies. However, a significant proportion of the British public opposes the use of animals in medical research.

The scale of animal experimentation in the UK

The number of animals used in medical research is small compared to the volume used in other areas:

- An estimated two million cats and dogs are abandoned as unwanted pets every year.

- Last year 800 million animals were slaughtered for human consumption.

- By contrast, only 2.6 million were used in medical research.[12]

The law

Animal experimentation is **governed by strict legislation.** Of all the areas in which animals are used (including agriculture, pets and sports), the required standards of welfare and veterinary care are the *highest* for laboratory animals. British legislation on the welfare of laboratory animals is among the strictest in Europe.

The Animals (Scientific Procedures) Act (1986) requires **licensing for all scientific procedures.** The Secretary of State decides whether to grant project licences by using a mainly utilitarian principle, weighing up the likely benefits of the research against the adverse effects on the animals used.

Ethical issues

Is it *right* to use animals for our own ends? What rights, if any, do animals have? And what duties, if any, do we owe them? The answers to these questions vary widely depending on our views on the moral status of animals and on the relationship between humans and animals.

Some key arguments in favour of, and against, animal research

- **Consequentialist arguments:**
FOR animal research: Throughout history, animal research has led to major advances in medicine. The use of animals in research produces a **huge benefit**. Not using animals will delay medical progress and result in much avoidable suffering.

Problems: How can we weigh up animal suffering against the potential gains of reducing human suffering? Is it right to use animals as means to our own end in this way, whatever the expected gains?

- **Moral status arguments:**

AGAINST: Arguments against the use of animals for research commonly focus on the **moral status** of animals.

Whether animals should be regarded as members of the moral community is controversial. Many people assess this by examining the qualities that the animals possess. At least some animals show '**indicators of humanhood**' (possessing distinct personalities, forming emotional attachments and passing on learned behaviours and customs through social mechanisms).[13]

Philosophers such as Peter Singer are more extreme, and argue that the **capacity to experience pain or pleasure** is the overriding qualification for membership of the moral community. If animals are part of this community, they should also benefit from the accompanying rights. But even if we accept that animals are sentient beings, or members of the moral community, it does not necessarily follow that they should have the same rights as humans.[14]

Problems: This type of argument can **raise awkward moral questions** if we accept that certain qualities dictate which beings are morally important. Some of these qualities are possessed by animals, but not by babies or brain damaged patients. Should we include a dog in the moral community but not a demented patient?[13]

IN FAVOUR: Although animals are morally important, the greater cognitive ability of humans gives them higher moral status. Therefore, it is justifiable to use animals to enhance human welfare.

> **Fun fact:** Legally, under the Treaty of Rome, animals are designated as '**agricultural products**' within the European Community. In 1991, a petition from the organisation *Compassion in World Farming* collected over 1 million signatures asking for their reclassification as sentient beings.[13]

- **Speciesist arguments:**

IN FAVOUR: Humans have greater moral status than animals by virtue of being a member of the human species.

AGAINST: As a superior species we are responsible for stewardship over other species. The concept of 'stewardship' does not necessarily include using animals for our own gains.

- **Disputed value argument:**

AGAINST: Some anti-vivisection organisations argue that animal-based research has contributed little to medical progress.[15] Conclusions from experiments can also be misleading. Animal research used for drug development has caused harm to humans through side effects.

Problems: Most of the evidence suggests that animal research has been of great value to humans. There is also a lack of viable alternative methods for the experiments currently carried out on animals.

Even if we conclude that animal experimentation may be morally acceptable (or even desirable), all would agree that research animals should be treated as humanely as possible. This entails minimizing the pain, distress and discomfort caused by experimental procedures. These aims are summed up by the 3Rs of Russell and Birch.[16]

The '3Rs' of using animals in research:

Replacement – replacing 'higher' animals (e.g. primates) with 'lower' animals (e.g. locusts) where possible, or finding new ways of doing things, such as using computer models.

Reduction – minimizing the number of animals used (i.e. using as few as possible to reach statistical significance. Avoiding unnecessary duplication of studies.)

Refinement – refining experimental protocols to minimize pain or distress whenever possible (e.g. using anaesthetics and analgesia). Properly trained staff to carry out procedures.

Summary

- Doctors have a duty to promote and encourage medical research.

- Medical research requires valid informed consent and good professional regulation to avoid the repetition of past abuses and to reassure the public.

- **Ethics committees** are the main form of regulation.

- There is a need to include a **wide variety of subjects,** without discriminating against certain groups.

- Research should meet a number of **strict criteria** to safeguard the welfare of participants, maintain public trust and ensure scientific validity. Requirements for innovative treatment are currently less stringent.

- Even with informed consent, the **duty of care rests with researchers** and expected harms to participants should be minimal.

- Special considerations apply to vulnerable groups such as children and those unable to consent for themselves.

- Animal research is a morally contentious, but strictly legislated area.

References

1. United States Holocaust Memorial Museum. The doctors trial. URL: www.ushmm.org/research/doctors/twoa.htm.

2. The Declaration of Helsinki is available online: www.wma.net/e/policy/b3.htm.

3. *Department of Health. Research governance framework for health and social care.* London, 2001.

4. Nicholson R. Final act in the Evelyn Thomas case. *Bulletin of Medical Ethics* 1992;75:3-4.

5. Home hazards injure thousands. *BBC News* 2001 7 June.

6. Hope T, Savulescu J, Hendrick J. *Medical ethics and law:* the core curriculum. Edinburgh: Churchill Livingstone, 2003.

7. British Medical Association; Medical Ethics Today. London: BMJ Publishing Group, 2004.

8. General Medical Council. The role and responsibilities of doctors.

9. Lock S. Editorial. Lessons from the Pearce affair: handling scientific fraud. *British Medical Journal* 1995;310:1547.

10. Wakefield A, Murch S, Anthony A, Linnell J, Casson D, Malik M, et al. Ileal-lymphoid-nodular hyperplasia, non-specific colitis, and pervasive developmental disorder in children. *The Lancet* 1998;351:637-641.

11. Giles J. Media attack prompts editorial backlash against MMR study. *Nature* 2004;427:765.

12. Seriously Ill for Medical Research website. URL: www.simr.org.uk/pages/research/.

13. Greyson L. *Animals in research: for and against*. London: British Library, 2000.

14. Singer P. *Animal liberation*. 2nd ed. London: Jonathan Cape, 1990.

15. The National Antivivisection Society. URL: www.navs.org.

16. Russell W, Birch R. *The principle of humane experimental technique*. London: Methuen, 1959.

Fetuses, aliens and violinists: human reproduction

The Embryo and the Fetus

The moral status of the embryo and fetus is central to the heated debate on abortion. One major disagreement between so-called pro-life advocates and pro-choice advocates is one of **scope:** does the moral norm forbidding the killing of innocent persons include the fetus? Put simply, 'pro-lifers' say fetuses should be included in the scope of the norm, whereas 'pro-choicers' believe fetuses lie outside the scope. We will examine the link between the moral status of the fetus and the various positions on abortion later. First, let us consider the legal status of the embryo and fetus.

The law on the fetus

- By law, an embryo or fetus is **not** a person. It does not have any legal rights. You cannot be charged with murder for killing a fetus, even if you kill it one minute before birth! It is only **at birth** that a fetus acquires all the legal rights (as long as it is born alive). This is why doctors who perform late term abortions try their best to kill the fetus *in utero*.

- A competent, pregnant mother can refuse treatment, **even if this entails the certain death of her fetus**.

Despite the above, the law does consider fetal interests in other ways:

- In theory, there is no abortion on demand. Certain criteria must be met for abortion to be legal, even for early term abortions.

- There are legal restrictions on the use of embryos in research.

The ethics

What the law considers acceptable is not necessarily *ethically* acceptable. Most people are appalled at the idea of a heavily pregnant mother smoking three packs of cigarettes a day, eating Big Mac meals for breakfast, lunch and dinner, drinking a bottle of whisky each evening, and training to be a full-contact kickboxer, but the law does not prohibit this. **A mother has no legal duty towards her unborn child.** Most people, however, believe a mother has *moral* duties towards her fetus.

Sometimes the law does not prohibit actions which most people find objectionable on the grounds that banning the action would cause more harm than good, or that the law would be too hard to enforce. Think of adultery, for example. No one thinks adultery is a good thing, but there are no laws against it.

In the case of allowing women to refuse treatment at the risk of killing the fetus, one possible reasoning behind the law is that it is wrong to force a woman to undergo surgery or some other medical procedure for the sake of another person, even if this might save that person's life. Respecting the autonomy of the mother, even if she is carrying an unborn child, is of such paramount importance that it trumps any *prima facie* duties towards the fetus. For some, the fetus should not be considered a 'person', since it has no autonomy. It does not have the cognitive faculties required to be a 'person'. For others, the ethical tension between the duties to the mother and the duties to the unborn child is much stronger and should not always be resolved in favour of the mother.

Parental obligations to a fetus

Although not required by law, it seems reasonable to attribute some **moral obligations** to pregnant mothers. These obligations would ensure that the mother does not harm the unborn child and avoids activities, such as boozing and kick-boxing, which would endanger the fetus. To use the language of virtue theory, a kind, considerate, caring, and responsible mother would most certainly fulfil these parental obligations. Only a vicious mother would knowingly do things that would harm her unborn child. The precise nature of these obligations, however, is open to debate.

What constitutes a 'person'?

As John Harris writes, if some odd-looking, extra-terrestrial creature landed on earth from outer space, how should we decide in which sense to 'have it for dinner'?[1] Should we invite the alien back to our place for a cuppa or should we shove it in the oven with two cloves of garlic and a dash of olive oil?

Below is a short list that might distinguish a person from a non-person:

* Consciousness.

- Ability to reason and reflect.

- Ability to communicate and interact in a meaningful way.

- Ability to consider one's own past and future.

- Ability to feel pleasure and pain, happiness and despair.

Perhaps what constitutes a person is not one, but a **combination** of these properties. In any case, it is not entirely clear what properties are required to call something a 'person'.

Even if we determined that our visiting alien was a person, it may still be acceptable to kill it in certain circumstances. Consider the following scenario:

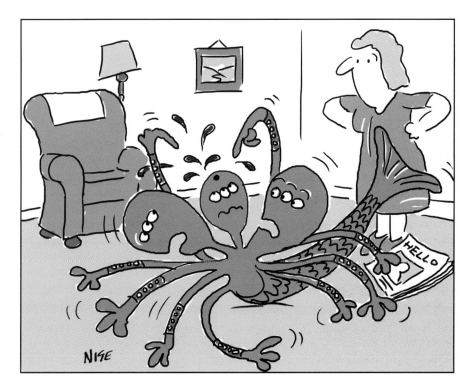

After pressing a few buttons on one of his many limbs, the alien suddenly talks English. Without doubt, he is a self-aware, reflective person...and a friendly one too! As he 'walks' towards you to greet you, he slips on an issue of Hello magazine which you inadvertently left on your living room floor. He crashes to the ground with a thump. The smallest of this three heads is oozing orange fluid. The alien, visibly shaken, tells you that he has lost so much vital fluid that he will self-destruct in a few seconds, killing all around him. The only way to prevent the explosion is to 'deactivate' the alien by removing the mole-like growth on his central head. The alien's communication system is down and, rather strangely, his body is inflating at an alarming rate. What should you do?

In this scenario, although the alien is an innocent person who wishes you no harm, many people would find it morally acceptable to deactivate the alien. Whether or not he intends to harm you, his presence is clearly life-threatening. Transferring this reasoning to the case of abortion, aborting fetuses which may cause life-threatening or very serious injury to the mother may be acceptable. The act is made in self-defence, as a last resort.

Killing the fetus/alien because it is merely inconvenient, however, would be morally wrong if we give the fetus/alien the same moral status as an adult human. But what do we mean by 'moral status'?

What is moral status?

A 'person', by most definitions, is a being with high moral status. When we attribute moral status to something, we acknowledge that it has a certain **moral standing**. We cannot just treat it as a mere object. **We have moral obligations towards it.**

The computer I am currently using, for example, has no moral status. I clumsily hit the keys with no remorse or guilt. I can smash the screen and pour hot coffee all over it and no one will say that I morally wronged the computer. I, however, have considerable moral status. In normal circumstances, if someone smashed my fashionable glasses and poured hot coffee all over me, they will have morally wronged me.

Note that moral status, like autonomy, can be present in different degrees. A garden slug may have some moral status (by virtue of being alive and possibly feeling rudimentary pain) but certainly not as much as a cat, which in turn won't have as much moral status as a human being.

Moral status is a **protective concept** which prevents us from treating things in any way we wish. If something has moral status, we have obligations to do or not do certain things to it. The strength of these obligations depends on how much moral status we give the entity. We can see why the question of whether a fetus has moral status – and, if so, how much – is crucial to the abortion debate! If it has 'full' moral status (i.e. as much as you or me), then killing the fetus could be viewed as murder. If it has no or very low moral status, then killing it is either indifferent or trivial.

Argument from potential

It is possible to say that a fetus has low current moral status while claiming that it is still wrong to kill it because of its *potential* to become a person with full moral status. The common counter-argument to this is to say that, with the advent of cloning, all somatic cells have the potential to become persons. Is killing a cell morally wrong? If so, we are all terrible people! We all scratch ourselves from time to time. Furthermore, the fact that X has a potential to be Y does not mean that it should enjoy the same rights and privileges as Y. You are all potential consultant cardio-thoracic surgeons, but no one claims you should prescribe drugs to severely ill patients, perform complex heart procedures, and do other things that surgeons do!

There are more sophisticated versions of the argument from potential, but we will not discuss these here. They can be found in the medical ethics literature.[2, 3]

How do we decide what has moral status?

The philosopher Mary-Anne Warren has come up with seven principles of moral status. The principles are criteria for assessing moral status and may help us decide in which way to have the alien 'for dinner'.

Much can be said about each of these but, for our purposes, we will simply list them and provide a short description of each.

1. **Respect for life principle** – don't kill living things unless you have good reason to do so.

2. **Anti-cruelty principle** – don't inflict pain on beings who can suffer.

3. **Agent's rights principle** – moral agents have equal rights, including the right to life and freedom.

4. **Human rights principle** – humans who can feel pain but have no agency (i.e. who don't have the capacity to evaluate their actions) have the same moral rights as other moral agents. This gives mentally disabled adults and children higher status than they otherwise would have.

5. **The ecological principle** – even if they have no agency or cannot feel pain, living things that are ecologically important have higher status that their intrinsic properties suggest. This provides a reason not to wipe out thousands of plant species to build a new Starbucks in Brazil.

6. **The interspecific principle** – animals that have close ties to the human community have higher moral status than their intrinsic properties suggest. Examples would be cows in parts of India and household pets in this country.

7. **The transitivity of respect principle** – moral agents should respect the decisions of others to give things moral status. For example, if I give my beloved garden slug, Sue, high moral status (it sleeps in my bed, watches TV with me, and joins me at the all-you-can-eat salad bar when I visit Pizza Hut), other people should respect my decision to give it higher moral status than they would.

Of course, these principles may conflict. The Agent's Rights Principle may require violating another principle, for example. For most people, there are times when killing a sentient being is not morally wrong, as in the case of self-defense. In cases of conflict, the moral agent will have to balance the principles in light of the specific context.

Abortion

What is the law on abortion?

The law on abortion is set out below (Abortion Act 1967, amended 1990).

Under 24 weeks, a doctor can perform an abortion if:

a) continuing the pregnancy poses a risk (greater than not being pregnant) of '*injury to the physical or mental health of the pregnant woman or any existing children of her family*' *and*

b) two registered doctors allow the abortion

Over 24 weeks, the conditions are much more stringent:

a) the abortion is needed to prevent '*grave permanent injury* to the physical or mental health of the woman', or

b) continuing the pregnancy would *put the woman's life at risk*, more so than not continuing the pregnancy, or

c) there is a '*substantial risk*' that the resulting child would suffer from physical or mental abnormalities that would make him *seriously disabled* (this is the most common reason for late-term abortions). What qualifies as 'substantial risk' is not made clear.

Conscientious objection

A doctor can refuse to perform an abortion if this goes against his conscience, except in an emergency (i.e. the mother would die or suffer serious mental or physical injury without an abortion).

> **Important note:** in an emergency, the opinion of a second doctor is not needed.
>
> **Another important note:** the biological father of the fetus cannot prevent the woman from having an abortion, nor can he force her to have one.

The objecting doctor must **explain** why he refuses to perform the procedure and **promptly refer** the patient to someone likely to perform the abortion.

Note that medical students can also have a conscientious objection to watching abortions. If this is the case, you should contact your clinical tutor.

Common positions on abortion

There are three major positions on abortion. Below each one, we have included a short summary of the argument and a few comments.

a) The **Human Being Argument** (the traditional pro-life position)

Premises:

1. It is wrong to *deliberately* kill an innocent (i.e. non-threatening) human being.

2. A fetus is an innocent human being.

therefore

Conclusion:

3. Deliberately killing a fetus is wrong.

Comments:

The fetus can, in some cases, threaten the mother's life. In this case, abortion would presumably be acceptable.

The argument refers to the 'deliberate' killing of the fetus. In some cases, doctors claim that they do not *deliberately* kill the fetus but that it is a foreseen side-effect of another procedure, such as removing a woman's uterus to treat a carcinoma. They appeal to the **doctrine of double effect** (see box below).

The Doctrine of Double Effect
As the name suggests, the doctrine says that it is morally acceptable to bring about a bad effect when intending to bring about a good effect as long as:

1. The intention is to bring about the good effect, not the bad effect (although the bad effect can be foreseen).

2. The intended good effect outweighs the bad effect (i.e. there must be a good enough reason to permit the bad effect to happen).

---

3. The good effect is actually good.

4. The good effect must not be achieved by bringing about the bad effect.

One good thing about the doctrine:
- It **highlights the importance of intention** in the morality of an act (and recognises that consequences are not everything).

A few bad things:
- **Intention versus foresight** – It can be very difficult to distinguish what is intended from what is foreseen. The philosopher Kamm gives the example of the terrorist who only intends innocent civilians to *appear* dead (so that the enemy will surrender) although he foresees that this will entail their actual death.[4] In hard cases, there is a certain fuzziness between what is intended and what is foreseen. Most of the time, however, the distinction is obvious, as when a surgeon foresees the possibility of death during an anaesthetic.

- **Proving intention** – How can we prove that a doctor's intention was to alleviate the cancer patient's pain with high doses of morphine rather than to kill the patient?

- **Absolutist element** – According to the theory, some acts are always wrong, even if they bring about great consequences. So, killing one evil dictator to save millions of children from torture would be wrong, because it would entail bringing about a good effect through a bad effect. The doctrine has an **absolutist** element to it (i.e. some acts are *always* wrong, irrespective of consequences). Many people disagree with this absolutist stance.

The doctrine of double effect in practice...
'Doctors are legally permitted to give sedatives and analgesics to sick patients with the intention of, and in proportion to, the relief of suffering, even if as a consequence the patient's life may be shortened. The moral distinction is between intending and foreseeing the harm. The intention of giving the drugs is to relieve the pain and distress of a dying patient; the harmful, but unintended, effect is the risk of shortening life, which the doctor may foresee but not intend.' (BMA's handbook of ethics and law, p. 378)[5]

b) The **Person Argument** (the traditional pro-choice position)

<u>Premises:</u>

1. A fetus is <u>not</u> a person.

2. Only persons have moral status.

therefore

<u>Conclusion:</u>

3. A fetus has no moral status (hence it's not wrong to kill it!).

Comments: This argument raises the following, thorny questions which we touched upon earlier: what is a person? And do only persons have moral status? What is moral status?

This position may imply that babies or severely disabled adults are not persons either. If they are not, does that mean we can treat them like mere objects since they have no moral status?

c) The **Woman's Body Argument** (a feminist position)

<u>Premises:</u>

1. A fetus is part of a woman's body.

2. A woman can do what she wants to her body.

Therefore

<u>Conclusion:</u>

3. A woman has a right to kill a fetus located inside her body.

Comments: The argument sidesteps the debate over the moral status of the fetus. Even *if* a fetus has a right to life, it does not have a right over the woman's body (see Thomson's violinist example below).

> **Thomson's violinist analogy**
> You wake up one day in hospital. In the bed next to you lies a world famous violinist, who is connected to you through all kinds of tubes and machines. You soon realise that you have been kidnapped by the Music Appreciation Society who, aware of the maestro's impending but preventable death from a rare kidney disease, hooked you up to the violinist. No one else can save him. In 9 months, the violinist will be cured and you will be free to go. Until then, however, you must stay in hospital.[6]

The story represents pregnancy, where a mother is 'stuck' with a fetus for 9 months. Without the mother's cooperation, the fetus will die. Thomson argues that you have no moral obligation to stay connected to the violinist for 9 months. You could if you wanted, and that would be jolly nice of you, but there is no moral obligation to do so. By analogy, a pregnant mother does not have a moral *obligation* to be pregnant for 9 months for the sake of the baby, even if this will result in the baby's death.

There are limits, however, to what we can do with our bodies and our property. I can't take a nap in the middle of a busy road, for example. Our freedom is constrained by other factors. So, in the case of a pregnant woman, someone might say that "yes, usually, a woman has right over her body, but not when there's a fetus in there!".

In short, the validity of Thomson's argument is based on a **theory of rights** that justifies acts by appealing to rights, whatever the consequences of the acts. Obviously, this would be denied by our friend Kevin the consequentialist. He would say that we should stay connected to the violinist if, after consideration, this is likely to lead to more overall good than overall harm. Some consequentialists would therefore reject Thomson's argument for abortion.

Note also that Thomson's analogy **only refers to accidental pregnancy or rape** (i.e. you did not want to be kidnapped and connected to the violinist).

One possible approach to abortion: the gradualist position

This position holds that the embryo or fetus gains in moral status as the pregnancy advances. This may be explained by the evolving development of the fetus, the tighter bond between mother and unborn child, or the increasing likelihood of the fetus to become a 'person'. Therefore, the required justifications for abortion also become more stringent as the weeks go by. The justifications needed to abort a fetus a day before birth will need to be much stronger than those needed to abort a 1-day-old embryo.

Using tissue from aborted fetuses

- Research on embryos is only allowed up to 14 days after fertilization (when the 'primitive streak' appears).

> **Note:** Embryos for research come from either IVF procedures (i.e. extra embryos which would either be discarded or given to other infertile couples) or from research, where they are specifically created.

- It is illegal to:

  a) create embryos by mixing human and animal gametes.

  b) create genetically identical individuals by genetic replacement (i.e. cloning).

  c) store embryos for more than 10 years.

- All research using fetal material must be reviewed by a Research Ethics Committee.

Is research on embryos or embryonic tissue ethical?

It depends, in part, on your views on the moral status of the embryo. If you give embryos full moral status, using them for research is unlikely to be ethical, even if the potential benefits to others are considerable.

For those who believe consequences are important (although not necessarily *all-important*, as consequentialists believe) in assessing the morality of an act, the likely benefits of the research are crucial. Also, the source of the embryos may be relevant. Some may not object to using surplus embryos from IVF but will be against deliberately creating embryos for research purposes. Dan the deontologist may invoke Kant's categorical imperative, enlarging the scope of the formula of humanity to include embryos (and not just rational, autonomous persons). On this view, using embryos solely as a means to an end would be morally wrong.

What benefits, if any, can be gained by using embryos in research?

When developing new infertility treatments, researchers must make sure the treatment will not damage the embryo or affect its development. This may require some embryos to be used as 'guinea pigs' to check that the technique is safe. Without these safeguards, the technique would either prove dangerous to the unborn child or would not be used at all.

Embryonic stem cells can be taken from embryos. As these stem cells can develop into any kind of cell, the therapeutic potential is enormous. They could be used to create skin for burn victims, muscle or neural tissue, or even bone marrow for those suffering from leukaemia.

Sterilisation

Sterilisation is a procedure that is likely to make the patient permanently infertile.

As for other medical procedures, the patient should give valid consent for the sterilisation. This requires a knowledge of the procedure itself, the likely side-effects, the alternative forms of contraception, and so on. The doctor should also ask the patient about the chances of her currently being pregnant and what to do if this turns out to be the case.

Although the decision to be sterilised ultimately rests with the individual patient, **patients should be encouraged to discuss this with their partners,** as the procedure has implications for them too!

Many people see sterilisation on competent adults as respecting autonomy, but some groups disapprove of the procedure. The Catholic Church considers sterilisation a form of bodily mutilation that goes against the natural function of humans to reproduce. Others believe that patients who ask for sterilisations are likely to change their minds later and will regret their decision.

Sterilising people with learning disabilities

The difference with severely mentally disabled people is that, unlike competent people, they do not possess **sufficient autonomy** to make a rational choice.

As they cannot always express their own wishes and values, balancing harms and benefits can prove difficult. The benefits can be more for the patients' carers, who may be tired of preventing the sexual escapades of their patients, than for the patients themselves. Remember that the treatment should be in the patient's best interests!

One way around the problem of insufficient autonomy: Ask 'what would the patient have wanted if autonomous now?' But what if he never was autonomous (e.g. disabled from birth) or if no one knows what he would have wanted?

Another way around it: use a proxy to decide on the patient's behalf. But what if the proxy is acting against the patient's best interests, or if there is no suitable proxy? Gillon gives three reasons why some people believe a proxy should not decide for an incompetent patient:[7]

1. It cannot be in a mentally disabled person's interests to be sterilised.

2. Sterilising a mentally disabled person without consent infringes their rights.

3. Sterilising mentally disabled persons goes against the interests of society (due to the anticipated harm to others or to the anticipated injustice).

Gillon counters each of these objections in the following way:

1. If it can be in a competent person's interests to be sterilised, can it not also be in a mentally disabled person's interests? **The benefit of the sterilisation is simply to avoid pregnancy.** In some cases, it is in the best interests of severely disabled persons to avoid pregnancy. Often, they will not be able to keep a child. If they are not sterilised, female patients will require either separation or constant supervision when around men. If they are sterilised, sexual interaction may be allowed.

   Some will say: "OK, but what about other, less drastic, types of contraception?" This is valid only if there is a **realistic chance for the patient to nurture a child later.** Also, it might be difficult for patients to safely use condoms or pills. More permanent types of contraception (e.g. intra-uterine device) have associated risks.

2. The patient's right to reproduction (or to have sex) is supposedly violated. It is generally accepted that surgery, if it is deemed in the patient's best interests, can be performed on an incompetent patient. What is the difference here? Furthermore, sterilisation does not infringe the 'right' to have sex, but promotes it!

3. Slippery slope: 'this might lead to the kind of mass sterilization seen in Nazi Germany'. Unlike the sterilisations done during the Nazi period, the sterilisations are **allowed only in the interests of the individual concerned,** not others. The approval of independent ethics committees can provide additional safeguards against the slippery slope argument (see box below).

The slippery slope argument
The argument, often used in medical ethics, goes like this: you should not allow A because if you allow A then B will happen and then C and so on all the way to E which is really bad. Therefore, don't allow A in the first place!

There are two types: **logical and empirical.**

The **logical slippery slope:** if you accept A, then you are *logically required* to accept B and *logically required* to accept C and so on, until you reach the evil E!

The *empirical slippery slope:* if you accept A, then you will *in all likelihood* accept B, and so on, until you reach the undesirable E.

Examples of the slippery slope argument
EMPIRICAL: there's *good evidence* to show that legalising morally acceptable cases of euthanasia will lead, through social and psychological processes, to legalising morally unacceptable cases of euthanasia (i.e. voluntary to non-voluntary to involuntary euthanasia).

Comment: you need to show the 'good evidence'!

LOGICAL: legalising suicide *logically entails* legalising voluntary euthanasia.

Comment: you need to show the logical entailment!

Note that the slippery slope argument can be used against anything than can be abused (e.g. ban electricity because terrorists use it to torture innocent people!).

Nevertheless, this does not mean that the argument itself is weak! Slippery slope arguments can be very strong.

For the slippery slope to be valid, you need to show that:

1   the bottom of the slope actually *is* bad!

2.   you cannot prevent the slide from A to E by putting in safeguards.

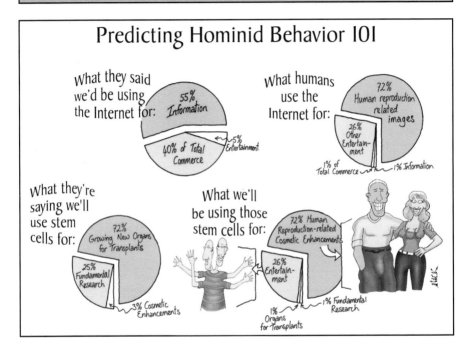

Three things to remember:

- Doctors should obtain valid consent before performing a sterilisation. They should mention side-effects, the difficulty of reversal and other, less permanent alternatives.

- Sterilisations should be done with the best interests of the patient in mind.

- The sterilisation of a mentally disabled person or a minor usually requires the permission of a High Court judge. Only when there are obvious medical benefits is judicial review not necessary.

Pre-natal screening and testing

Prenatal screening allows parents to know a lot about the health of their future baby. It can also bring them some **peace of mind** or, if things are not too rosy, it can give them time to mentally and practically **prepare themselves for the future.** For the medical team too, it can give them **advance warning** on what the delivery will require and what treatment, if any, will be needed.

Although prenatal screening is recommended for mothers at higher risk of giving birth to a disabled child, such as injecting drug users, the doctor should still obtain the woman's consent.

As prenatal testing can identify unborn children with a genetic condition, it is offered to mothers who have a family history of a particular disease or who have had previous pregnancies with an affected child. Again, even if there is a very high probability of a serious inheritable disease, the woman's consent should be obtained.

If parents disagree over whether to have a test, the doctor should encourage them to talk it over to arrive at a mutually acceptable solution. If the couple disagree, the law says that the **mother's wish is trumps!**

What kind of ethical issues are there in pre-natal testing and screening?

There can be an ethical tension between the wishes of the mother (principle of respect for autonomy directed at the mother) and the welfare of the future child (principles of beneficence and non-maleficence directed at the unborn child). The mother's refusal to undergo prenatal tests may result in the birth of a severely disabled child. If we believe that a mother has parental obligations even during her pregnancy (which prohibits her to drink, smoke and take up kung-fu), then these obligations may well include taking tests to rule out serious disability.

One could argue that even severely disabled fetuses should not be aborted by using the following argument: if X, a fetus who will develop a serious disability, is aborted, then X will no longer exist. Unless X's quality of life will be so awful that it would be better for X not be born at all (e.g. the baby suffers from anencephaly or Tay-Sachs disease), then it is in X's interests to carry on living. A life worth living must surely be preferable to non-existence. However, even if we accept this argument (and there are several objections to it), pre-natal testing could still be useful in preventing the birth of babies with conditions so terrible that life would be a curse rather than a blessing.

Some people who are against prenatal screening claim that such screening **expresses a disrespectful attitude towards the disabled,** as it suggests that disabled persons are unwanted. A common counter-argument to this objection (which is often referred to as the **expressivist objection**) is that it is not the *people* with disabilities that are disvalued or disrespected but the *disabilities* themselves.

Another counter-argument is to say that mere offense does not mean we should give up the opportunity to reduce or prevent human suffering.

Yet another objection to prenatal diagnosis is to say that it is 'unnatural'. But what do we mean by natural or unnatural? Can human inventions not be considered 'natural'? Why are we different from the rest of nature? Besides, all of medicine can be said to be interfering with nature. Think of vaccinations or surgery! In fact, think of umbrellas – should we not use them because they are unnatural?

Criteria for prenatal diagnosis

Imagine that prenatal diagnosis reveals a rare genetic condition that is invariably fatal at age 30. Should the mother be offered an abortion? If so, should the mother accept it? What if a mother wants to use the procedure to ensure that her future child has certain physical characteristics? Is it ethically acceptable for the technology to be used not just to reduce suffering but to 'enhance' people too?

These are incredibly difficult questions. People may have different views on these issues, as well as sound reasons to support their position. For exam purposes, the important thing is to articulate those reasons and to have strong justifications for the position taken.

When is prenatal diagnosis appropriate?

Again, there is no simple answer to this question. The BMA has come up with factors to consider when deciding on the appropriateness of prenatal diagnosis. (p. 254)[5]

These are:

• The sensitivity and specificity of the test and its level of predictability.

• The woman's own perception of the situation and her current family situation.

• The severity of the disorder and the age of onset.

• The available options, including possible treatment either in the womb or after birth.

Assisted conception

Assisted conception is a general term referring to the methods used to assist a woman conceive a child when she unable to do so by 'natural' means.

Interesting Fact: 1/10 couples are infertile and 1/6 have trouble conceiving.

For ease of reference, we have compiled a list of questions and answers relating to assisted conception.

Who can donate gametes?

Not everyone can donate their gametes for use in assisted conception. Certain conditions must first be met:

• Sperm donors must be under 45. Egg donors under 35.

• Fertility centres should check a prospective donor's medical history for genetic disorders, transmissible diseases, and potential fertility. They should also ask prospective donors why they wish to donate and whether they have any children.

• Couples where the woman is over 35 and the man over 45 can only have their gametes taken if these are used on themselves. They should be offered advice and counselling about the treatment.

Who can have IVF treatment?

• If a centre refuses to offer treatment to a couple, they must explain their refusal. The reason would usually be that the couple is **medically unsuitable** or that it would **not be in the future child's best interests**.

• The welfare of the future child and existing children must be considered before offering treatment.

• The clinic should also consider:
  – Why the couple want a child.
  – The environment in which the child will live.
  – The health and age of the parents and the relevance of these factors to their ability to deal with a child.
  – What happens if there are multiple births.
  – The risk of harm to the child.
  – The impact of the child on existing children.

• The centre must consider, in advance, the legal implications of the procedure, such as who will be legally responsible for the child.

Can people find out if they were born using assisted conception?

Yes, once a person reaches 18, they can ask the HFEA if they were born through assisted conception. Once a person reaches 16, they can ask the HFEA if their potential marriage partner is related to them! The HFEA keeps a record of all births resulting from fertility treatment.

Can people use their dead partner's gametes to conceive a child?

It depends. Partners may consent **in writing** to have their gametes stored so that their partner could conceive at a later date. If specific consent is not given, retrieving gametes from a dead spouse is generally unethical.

Is pre-implantation genetic diagnosis legal in the UK?

Pre-implantation genetic diagnosis (PGD) is **permitted only on medical grounds**. Sex selection, unless for medical purposes, is thus prohibited.

Can older women have IVF?

Again, it depends on the circumstances. Clinics are required by law to consider the **welfare of the future child and existing children**. For post-menopausal women, the HFEA states that decisions should be made on a case-by-case basis. If the parents can look after the child in a safe environment and other important criteria are met, providing treatment for older women may be acceptable.

Note also that fertility clinics should offer counselling to anyone wanting fertility treatment.

> **An ethical objection**
> Some people believe that all these constraints for allowing assisted reproduction discriminates against infertile people. After all, some say, we allow fertile, inconsiderate, alcoholic, drug-taking idiots to freely reproduce so why should we be so cautious just because a couple is infertile? One response is to say that since doctors are directly involved in the treatment, they have a duty to consider the welfare of the future child. As soon as a third party is involved, that party must ensure that they fulfil their own moral duties.

Although assisted conception is legal in the UK, some people are strongly against the practice. Most of them use one or both of these objections:

* Killing embryos is wrong (creating surplus embryos is a necessary byproduct of the procedure). *This depends on the moral status you give the embryo.*

* Assisted conception is unnatural and offensive. It is also 'playing God'. *Offensiveness, however, is not in itself unethical. Today, for example, I (DKS) joined a gym. When the time came to shower, I realised, to my considerable embarrassment, that I had only brought a small hand towel. Due to the towel's size, I had to hold it together around my waist when walking in the changing room. Although some people, no doubt, were amused by this risible sight, others may well have been offended. Yet their offence does not mean that I acted unethically. Offensiveness, in itself, is not morally wrong.*

The article below examines the perils of relying solely on our 'yuk' response.

Article: Reflecting on your 'yuk'

In April 2004, Julia Black's documentary 'My fetus' showed an abortion for the first time on British television. With a swoosh and a spurt of blood, the vacuum pump sucked out the 4-week-old foetus from the womb. In the closing months of 2003, transplant surgeons in Britain, France and the United States declared themselves ready to graft the face of a corpse onto a living recipient. In January 2004, Armin Meiwes, the 'German cannibal', was cleared of murder for killing and eating Bernd Brandes, a 43-year-old engineer who freely offered his life and flesh to satisfy Meiwes' unusual appetite. That same month, a renowned bioethicist suggested that infanticide may be acceptable. At first sight, these events are worthy of the most gruesome horror film. They engender a powerful sense of revulsion, an immediate 'yuk' response. For some, however, these acts may not be morally wrong at all. So who is right? And what should we make of this familiar 'yuk' response?

Recently, a highly respected bioethicist argued that infanticide may, in limited circumstances, be justifiable. According to him, it may be morally desirable to kill a baby if it is severely disabled or premature. Yuk! Killing babies is morally hideous, let alone illegal. Julia Millington, the political director of the ProLife party, called such a suggestion 'absolutely horrifying'. Clearly, obviously, undeniably, the bioethicist is wrong.

In a time when we are bombarded with bizarre stories, many of us rely on this intuitive response to form opinions on new ideas and technologies. But, on reflection, where is the argument behind our 'yuk' response? Expressing horror is not, in itself, a valid argument. It is merely displaying a disapproving attitude. 'I don't like it' may be a good reason when choosing your favourite colour, but it is not enough when discussing the morality of abortion or face transplants. The bioethicist's view cannot be dismissed solely on the basis of our repugnance.

History is strewn with examples of misplaced disgust. When chloroform was first used in the 19th century, relieving patients from the excruciating and often life-threatening pain of surgery, many people vigorously protested against the satanic invention. Since God inflicted disease as a punishment for our sins, any attempt to remove the pain was deemed blasphemous. Besides, chloroform was profoundly unnatural, the dissenters argued. Similar arguments were used to criticize the advent of *in vitro* fertilization in the late 1970s. When, in 1968, the first successful heart transplant took place in South Africa, thousands of people gasped 'yuk' in horror, not at the idea of transferring someone's heart into another's body, but at the colour of the donor's skin. That a white person should receive a black man's heart was repulsive to many. Countless other now common procedures also generated 'yuk' responses in the past.

These examples from history show the evolution of what society considers permissible. They also illustrate the danger of our 'yuk' responses. However powerfully felt, they can reflect prejudice and ignorance. They can blind us from the real reasons behind our objections, preventing all attempts at reflection. It is a mistake to rely on our gut feeling alone when assessing the morality of an act. Instead, this 'yuk' response should force us to think hard about *why* necrophilia, which has recently been made illegal in the UK, is undesirable, or why killing disabled babies is wrong or why eating people is immoral, even if they want to be devoured!

'Man is a credulous animal, and must believe *something*' wrote the philosopher Bertrand Russell 'in the absence of good grounds for belief, he will be satisfied with bad ones'. In an age of consensual cannibalism, Frankenstein foods, cloning and other peculiar scenarios, our gut reactions must be followed by a more composed phase of questioning and reasoning. Even if we staunchly disagree with an idea, a technology, or a new medical procedure, we must embrace the opportunity to reflect on our own position and not hide behind the treacherous comfort of 'yuk!'.[8]

Sex selection

As we mentioned earlier, sex selection is currently illegal in the UK, unless for serious sex-linked genetic diseases. Nevertheless, there is an ongoing ethical debate about whether it should be permitted for non-medical reasons, such as family balancing.

There are two separate questions to consider:

1. is it morally wrong to select a child's sex?

2. should be it legal?

When assessing the morality of an act, it is always a good idea to look at the **motives and attitudes** underlying the decision to act:

- If someone wants sex-selection because they think girls are inferior, then this is clearly an objectionable attitude.

- But what if someone with four boys wants their fifth child to be a girl? There is arguably less to object about in this case. So wanting sex selection for family balancing reasons is quite different from wanting the procedure because you think girls are evil.

What are the arguments AGAINST sex selection?

Here are some common arguments against sex selection, with some accompanying comments.

- *Sex selection is a misallocation of resources.* Not if it is done privately. If that is the case, some will complain that only the rich will be able afford it. You could then point to cosmetic surgery, which is also beyond the means of most people. Justice does not require total equality of access to healthcare but, more plausibly, to a minimum standard of healthcare (unless you're a strict egalitarian).

- *Sex selection is using a child to fulfil a couple's own desires* (hence violating Kant's dictum never to treat people only as means but also as ends). This also true of non-selected children! Few children are born purely as ends. Most parents have expectations regarding their children (for example, to provide company to an existing child)

- *Sex selection harms the child.* This is unlikely in our society, where girls and boys have pretty much equal status. Furthermore, some could claim that the particular child would not have existed without the procedure, so it has no grounds for complaint.

- *Sex selection is wrong per se – it is unnatural or 'playing God'!* But, again, so is most of medicine. There is also a potential **inconsistency,** since few people complain about other methods of sex-selection (such as conceiving close to ovulation, altering one's diet, trying different sexual positions, and so on).

The main reason for *allowing* sex selection is that it respects the **reproductive liberty** of women, such as the freedom to have children, to choose how many children to have, and with whom. But **not all liberties are absolute.** As we saw in earlier chapters, there are times when it is wrong to respect people's autonomy.

1. **Respect for autonomy may interfere with the basic liberties of others.** Selecting sex doesn't appear to violate the liberties of others, so we must look at the reasons below.

2. Reproductive decisions may be harmful to the child or mother.

3. **Legalising** sex selection may have broader **social costs.**

So, to convincingly show that sex selection is bad, you need further argument. You may want to show, for example, that the possible consequences of sex selection are bad. You can appeal to sexual justice (e.g. it will devalue women), an uneven sex ratio with undesirable consequences, or even formulate a slippery slope argument (e.g. if you allow people to select for sex, then why not for eye colour, intelligence...all the way to Nazi-style eugenics!). You might want to argue that the techniques for selecting sex, such as sperm sorting, are currently unsafe. You may find some of these reasons persuasive, or you may disagree with them. In either case, you must have good reasons to support your position.

Summary

- By law, the **fetus has no legal rights** until birth.

- A woman can refuse treatment, *even if* this entails the death of her unborn child.

- A pregnant mother may have **moral duties** towards her unborn child, even though there are no legal duties.

- Moral status is a **protective concept** that prevents us from treating things in any way we like.

- The requirements for obtaining an abortion differ significantly **before 24 weeks** and **after 24 weeks.**

- There are three main positions on abortion: **the human being argument, the person argument and the woman's body argument.**

- The **doctrine of double effect** states that it may be OK to bring about a bad effect when intending to bring about a good effect, as long as certain conditions are met.

- Research on embryos is allowed **up to 14 days after fertilization.**

- There are two types of slippery slope argument: **logical** and **empirical.**

- The mother's **consent** is required for pre-natal screening and testing.

- Revulsion ('yuk!') is not, in itself, a sufficient reason to label something as morally wrong.

References

1. Harris J. The concept of the person and the value of life. *Kennedy Institute of Ethics Journal* 1999;9(4):293-308.

2. Marquis D. A future like ours and the concept of person: a reply to McInerney and Paske. In: Pojman L, Beckwith F, editors. *The abortion controversy:* a reader. 2nd ed. Belmont, CA: Wadsworth, 1998:372-385.

3. Boonin D. *A defense of abortion.* Cambridge: Cambridge University Press, 2003.

4. Kamm F. Non-consequentialism. In: LaFollette H, editor. *The Blackwell Guide to Ethical Theory.* Oxford: Blackwell Publishing, 2000:205-226.

5. British Medical Association; Medical Ethics Today. London: BMJ Publishing Group, 2004.

6. Thomson J. A defense of abortion. *Philosophy and Public Affairs* 1971;1:47066.

7. Gillon R. On sterilising severely mentally handicapped people. *Journal of Medical Ethics* 1987;13:59-61.

8. Sokol D. In medicine, 'yuk' is not a useful guide. *International Herald Tribune* 2004 18 May.

Genetic counselling and the "new genetics'

The expanding field of genetics holds great potential for improving health and eradicating disease. Already, we can check whether a child is likely to develop certain diseases before it is even born. More generally, scientists can clone and genetically manipulate all kinds of animals, creating frogs without heads or mice with human ears. In the future, as we unravel the genetics of common diseases, genetic technologies might give us accurate predictions of disease risk and allow us to tailor drugs to specific individuals.

Yet many people are concerned about the social and ethical implications of genetic knowledge and technology. Ethical issues surround both the 'new' genetic techniques of gene therapy and reproductive cloning, and the practice of genetic counselling in the clinic. In fact, genetics and ethics are so enmeshed that a new term has been coined: 'genethics'.

What is genetic counselling?

Genetic counsellors provide information to families affected by genetic disorders and help patients understand the available options. Genetic counselling may include:

- Giving patients information on their likelihood of **developing** a genetic disorder.

- Educating them about the possible **consequences** of the disorder. ie. Its effect on their lives.

- Discussing the likelihood of a couple passing it on to their children. This may include ways to **prevent transmission** of a disorder if the couple request it.

Genetic counselling is supposed to be **non-directive**, meaning that doctors *provide information* to allow patients to make their own choices, but avoid telling patients which options they *ought* to choose. There are several reasons why a non-directive approach might be appropriate in genetic counselling:

1. It enhances patient autonomy, by respecting the patient's own wishes and values.

2. The values of the treating doctor, or of the medical community in general, do not interfere with the patient's decision-making process.

3. The medical profession is not seen to pass judgement on which lives are worth living.

There may also be disadvantages to a non-directive approach:

1. It is **inconsistent** with most other areas of medical practice. Often, doctors do not just provide factual information. They also give advice on what they think the best options are.

2. Many patients **want and expect** their doctors to give them advice. Why should this be any different for consultations relating to genetic conditions?

3. Patients are more likely to make the 'wrong' decision based on false beliefs or a misunderstanding of information. For example, if a patient refuses life-saving treatment, the doctor is aware that the patient may be making the 'wrong' decision. The doctor can then find out the patient's reasons for the refusal and confirm that the decision was made on a true understanding of the risks. Misunderstandings or obviously 'wrong' decisions are arguably harder to detect with a non-directive approach.

4. The treating doctor may feel that he *does know* the 'best' course of action, but cannot share it with the patient.

Ethical issues in clinical genetics

What kind of ethical issues do clinical geneticists encounter? Many of their day-to-day concerns are no different to those in other areas of medicine. Issues of informed consent and patient confidentiality are particularly important in the genetic clinic. However, there is an *added dimension* to ethical issues in clinical genetics, stemming from the **familial nature** of genetic information. By its nature, genetic testing does not just provide information about the patient taking the test. It also reveals details about the genes of the patient's relatives.

If my father decides to undergo testing for Huntington's disease (a severe inherited neurodegenerative disorder), this could have a huge impact on me. If he tested positive, I would have a 50/50 chance of developing the fatal condition. I might not want to know that! Doctors thus need to be aware of the **interdependence of interests** within families. In fact, not just doctors, but patients too should be aware of these interests. We can argue that we *all* have a moral duty to consider the interests of our family.

Case one: the parent and child problem

John Brown is a young man whose **maternal grandfather** has **Huntington's disease.** This devastating disorder does not usually present until late middle age, by which time sufferers often have children of their own. It is inherited in an autosomal dominant manner with *complete penetrance* (i.e. if you inherit the gene, you will definitely develop the disorder).

John is currently 25 and is thinking about starting a family of his own. If his grandfather suffered from the disease, he knows he has a **1 in 4** chance of being affected himself. This will depend on whether or not his mother, Lynn, has inherited the gene expansion that causes Huntington's from her father.

John comes to the genetic clinic to ask for predictive testing. He also tells you that his mother is **opposed** to his decision to take the test. Lynn, who is 48, has always declined the chance of testing, as she does **not want to know** her status.

This poses a difficult ethical problem for the geneticist, since testing John also reveals Lynn's genetic status. Allowing John to exercise his right to know his genetic status appears to violate his mother's right not to know (if either of these rights exist!).

There is also a consent issue here, as 'essentially, the mother is receiving information about her health as if she had been tested without her consent'.(p. 315)[1] A similar situation occurs when the patient undergoing a test is one half of a monozygotic twin pair, and the other twin does not wish to know his genetic status.

What should you do about such cases in practice?

Doctors usually encourage patients who request genetic tests to **involve other family members** in the decision. In cases like that of the Brown family, you would ideally test the mother first, assuming she consented to the test and was happy to know her genetic status. But in some cases, as Lynn Brown did, the mother refuses the test. If so, what should you do about her son's request?

In practice, those at a 25% risk of Huntington's may be encouraged to think about whether they need to undergo testing at that *precise point* in time. The mother may well reconsider her decision in a few years. Alternatively, she might develop symptoms of the disease, revealing her status anyway. However, in practice, testing would **not be withheld** from John *solely* on the grounds that it would reveal information about his mother.

Case 2: family feuds and non-disclosure

Anne and Geoff are a couple that you saw regularly in the genetic clinic last year. Their son suffered from a rare **childhood genetic disorder** and died in infancy. A diagnosis was made on the basis of DNA testing, and the disorder was found to be an **X-linked condition.**

You now see **another branch** of the **same family** in the clinic. Anne's sister, Jane, is seeking advice as she is aware of a possible genetic disorder in the family. The sisters have not spoken for the past two years following a family row.

Jane asks you to establish if she carries the mutation that causes the condition. To do this, you need to know what the mutation is. You ask Anne for consent to release the DNA result to her sister. However, **she refuses,** claiming a right to her genetic privacy.

This is a tricky situation. Arguably, Jane could be harmed without this information. In these sorts of cases, the doctor faces a conflict between the duty to maintain patient confidentiality and the duty to protect others from avoidable harm.

In the field of clinical genetics, some argue that the doctor's 'patient' is not the isolated individual, but the **entire family unit.** The obligation of geneticists should thus extend beyond the individual to the relatives. According to this view, disclosing genetic information to other family members would *not constitute a breach of confidentiality.* This is a bold claim, which we shall not attempt to refute here. As far as the law is concerned, the duty of confidentiality remains to the **individual patient.** So, usually, you would have to respect Anne's wish to withhold the information from Jane.

The patient's confidentiality may be breached, however, in situations where doing so would be in the public interest (see chapter 4). For example, a patient might refuse to share information with a relative, who is then put at risk of a **severe but treatable life threatening disorder.**

Several factors might influence your decision to disclose the information to others:[1]

- How **severe** the resulting disorder might be.

- How **good** the test is at predicting whether others are at risk.

- What **actions** the relatives could take to protect themselves against the possible adverse effects of the disorder.

- Whether it is possible to **identify** the relatives without the assistance of the patient (i.e. if they are your patients, you have a duty of care towards them too).

To prevent such situations from arising, doctors routinely seek consent for sharing DNA results with certain relatives *before* testing. However, a refusal to consent should normally be respected. In practice, many patients later decide to release the information to other family members.

Informed consent for genetic testing

It is vital to provide clear information when consenting patients for genetic testing. You must ensure that patients understand what the result of the test will, and **will not** tell them. For example:

- Huntington's disease is one of the more straightforward examples, as this disease shows complete penetrance. **All patients** found to be carrying the gene expansion **will** develop the disease. However, we cannot give them a good estimation of **when** this will occur. It may happen within a few years, or in decades.

- For many other conditions, the uncertainty is even greater. For example, in the case of inherited breast cancer, the BRCA1 gene has *incomplete penetrance*. That means, that even if the genetic test is positive, the patient may not develop hereditary breast cancer.

- Does the patient understand the possible **adverse consequences** of an unfavourable test result? These are discussed further below.

- Have they made plans for what they will do if the result is positive? Has plenty of **support** and **follow-up** been arranged?

Why do patients want genetic testing?

Many patients at risk of a serious disease (such as Huntington's) decide that they don't want to know their genetic status. For those who **do** want to know, it is often useful to find out their **reasons** for wanting the test. As in any consultation, understanding the patient's concerns will help you give appropriate information and support.

There are several possible benefits of testing:

1. **Resolves uncertainty:** Many patients constantly worry about developing the condition. Their daily life may be disturbed by **intrusive thoughts** about the disease. For example, some individuals at risk of Huntington's disease worry every time they drop their keys or forget an item of shopping. They interpret these commonplace acts as the first step towards neurological decline.

2. **Allows planning:** Some patients may wish to alter their 'life plan' if they roughly know how many healthy years they have left. They may decide to steer clear of certain careers, such as medicine or law, which require many years of study, for example. Perhaps they will decide to travel the world instead. They can also sort out financial and other matters whilst they are still well.

3. Gives access to relevant **screening and preventive measures** if they exist (e.g. colonoscopy for hereditary bowel cancer). However, those with a family history of such conditions should have access to such screening even if they decide **not** to know their genetic status.

4. To **avoid passing on** a hereditary condition to children, or to allow the option of undergoing pre-natal testing if at risk.

As well as being beneficial, testing can also be harmful:

1. **Psychological harms:** patients can suffer from depression, anxiety and adjustment problems if they receive an unfavourable result.

2. **Financial harms:** patients may be unable to obtain life insurance, health insurance or a mortgage.

Insurance

Genetic testing can have major implications for a patient's ability to take out medical or life insurance. Many people believe insurance companies should not have access to genetic information, as this is unfair and constitutes a 'misuse' of personal information. But insurance companies currently have access to other medical information on potential clients. Certainly, patients have to disclose 'pre-existing' medical conditions, which are then excluded from cover. They may also have to undergo a medical examination. Why should the results of genetic tests be any different?

There are several arguments in favour of insurance companies having access to the results of genetic tests. If such results are known to the patient, but not to the insurer, the two parties are entering into an agreement based on **different levels of knowledge.** For example, the patient could take out a high value policy knowing that, in all likelihood, he will make a claim on it within a few years. This is unjust both to the insurance company and to its other customers, who will pay the cost in terms of higher premiums. There are also arguments against access. If those with unfavourable genetic test results are refused insurance cover, this might **deter** people from seeking genetic testing. This could result in some of the harms mentioned earlier.

At the moment, the situation with regards to insurance is rather complicated. The Government and the Association of British Insurers agreed on a **voluntary moratorium** on the use of predictive genetic testing until November 2006.[1] Patients do not have to disclose an 'unfavourable' test result to insurers. How valuable this is to patients is debatable. They may not have to disclose the actual test result, but they still have to disclose the *family history* of the condition. In practice, patients who receive a favourable result will usually choose to disclose it to insurers, as this increases their chances of obtaining insurance.

So it may be possible for insurers to infer a patient's genetic status from the fact that a) they have a positive family history, and b) they have not declared a favourable test result. Companies may load policies *as heavily* against patients on the basis of the family history as they would on the basis of a test result. At present, the debate continues about the fairest way to use genetic test results for insurance purposes.

Should we perform genetic testing on children?

Few contest that testing children for disorders that will affect them *during childhood* is acceptable. What is more controversial is the use of predictive testing for **adult-onset** conditions, or to determine whether children are carriers of certain conditions.

Arguments in favour of testing children:

• **Resolves uncertainty:** as for adults, this may reduce the anxiety and stress of not knowing for the child and the parents.

• **Allows informed decision-making:** this knowledge may affect the child's decisions about career plans, financial choices, relationships and having children.

• **Allows earlier adjustment:** gives more time to come to terms with things; the child can make his life plans around the knowledge.

• **Respects the autonomy of the child and the parents.**

Arguments against:

• **Fails to respect the child's autonomy:** early testing may violate the child's autonomy by denying him the chance *not* to know.

• **Possible harms to the child:** finding out about the diagnosis might have adverse consequences, especially if he does not fully understand the implications. There may be personal, financial, and psychological implications for the child and family. The parents may treat the child differently, for example.

In practice, it is **very rare** to perform predictive testing for adult-onset conditions in children, even if the parents request it. Families with children affected by a genetic disorder may also seek *carrier status* testing for their **unaffected** children. These requests are also unlikely to be granted. The main argument in support of not testing children is that testing violates a child's autonomy by removing his future right 'not to know' his genetic status. Testing may however be offered to **teenagers** if they are deemed (Gillick) competent to consent to the test.

Gene therapy

Gene therapy is a new technological process, which attempts to correct for defective genes that cause disease.[2] There are many ways to do this. Commonly, a 'normal' copy of the disease-causing gene is inserted into the genome using a viral vector. The Gene Therapy Advisory Committee (GTAC) oversees all gene therapy research in the UK. Currently, gene therapy research trials are restricted to patients suffering from **life threatening** disorders.

There are **two types** of gene therapy: somatic and germline:

Somatic:

• Produces genetic changes to somatic cells.

• Used to treat disease (or perhaps one day to enhance normal characteristics) in that individual patient only.

Germline:

• Induces genetic changes in gametes.

• Affects not only the patient himself, but also his descendents.

Ethical issues in gene therapy

A government committee which considered the ethics of **somatic** gene therapy concluded that it did *not* raise any particular new **ethical** challenges.[3] However, ongoing **safety** concerns have held back the introduction of gene therapy into clinical practice. Although gene therapy trials began in 1990, no gene therapy products have yet been licensed for clinical use. In 1999, an 18-year-old man died of multi-organ failure after only 4 days of treatment. He is thought to have suffered a severe immune response to the viral vector used.[4]

Germline gene therapy is more ethically contentious. Somatic gene therapy procedures affect only the individual patient. By contrast, germline therapy produces changes that will be passed on to future generations. This might be an advantage if the main use of gene therapy is to cure genetic disease. By repairing the faulty gene in the germ cell line, we abolish the need to repair the defect in every generation using somatic gene therapy. This maximises total welfare and is a more efficient, cost-effective way of achieving the same outcome as somatic gene therapy.[4]

However, there are also arguments against operating on the germline. Firstly, any *unforeseen* side effects of the manipulation might have a knock-on effect on successive generations. Secondly, the 'harmful' genes that we are altering or replacing may have *secondary functions* that would be beneficial in some environments. By altering the germline, these secondary functions would be lost forever.

The counter-argument to this is to say that even if this were true, using somatic rather than germline therapy would not prevent the loss of these secondary functions. If the original disease is sufficiently serious, sufferers would still want to opt for somatic gene therapy, whatever the possible 'secondary functions'. The only way to discover these secondary functions would be to leave a few 'guinea pigs' who would be denied gene therapy in each generation. The idea of untreated 'guinea pigs' is not an ethically appealing one!

There is widespread agreement that we should not be undertaking germline gene therapy at the present time. The objection is based primarily on safety concerns, rather than on any fundamental ethical difference between somatic and germline therapy. The Committee on the Ethics of Gene Therapy concluded that: '[there is] insufficient knowledge to evaluate the risks to future generations of gene modification of the germ line'.[3]

Some ethicists have an additional concern about gene therapy: that it might be used not just to treat the abnormal, but to **improve the normal.** In principle, it might be possible to target somatic gene therapy at muscle cells to make someone run faster, or at brain cells to make them more intelligent. Should we allow the genetic enhancement of natural abilities? The table below presents some common arguments for and against, as well as possible counter-arguments.

Arguments in favour	Counter-arguments
We already allow people to enhance their own talents and abilities through non-genetic means, e.g. education, specialist academies for athletes and musicians. Preventing enhancement through genetic means is thus **inconsistent.**	Genetic manipulations are permanent and dramatic. Unlike taking piano lessons or playing football, the individual would have no choice on the matter. Genetic enhancement might actually change the identity of the individual.
Distributive justice may require us to **correct** for the natural injustice of the distribution of talent. Some people are born clever, athletic and good-looking. Others, unfortunately, are dumb, scrawny and ugly. Is that fair?	Injustice could be corrected through **social means.** Indeed, genetic enhancement may even *increase* injustice, as perhaps only the rich would be able to afford it.
We should not restrict the **liberty** of individuals to act in the best interests of their children.	Restricting individual liberty may be justified in the wider public interest or to prevent deeply immoral acts.

Arguments against	Counter-arguments
Genetic enhancement is **eugenic**. Selecting out those characteristics thought to be 'unfavourable' (e.g. short sight, low intelligence) from the gene pool might eventually lead society to shun certain 'sub-standard' individuals.	We already try to improve health through medicine, surgery, and pre-implantation screening. When we use laser surgery to correct short sight, we are not implying that short-sighted individuals are *less worthy* than those with perfect refraction. Whether or not people are tolerant of a quality (e.g. blindness) does not necessarily depend on large numbers of individuals possessing that quality.

Arguments in favour	Counter-arguments
Genetic enhancement is **unnatural.**	The characteristics themselves are not unnatural as some members of the population already possess them! (unless we make people have wings or other unusual characteristics!) Even if enhancement is unnatural, it is not more so than the rest of medicine. And why can't we improve on the natural?
Enhancing individuals for 'desirable' traits (e.g. height, athleticism, intelligence) will result in a **loss of genetic diversity.**	The human genome contains over 100,000 genes, and enhancements would only involve a handful. Genetic enhancement will only affect a small percentage of the global population. Furthermore, there is no evidence that genetic diversity is necessary for human flourishing.
Adapted from Hope, Savulescu and Hendrick (2003),[5] and Harris (1998).[4]	

Practical problems

Even if (and it's a big 'if') we decide that it is morally desirable to use gene therapy to produce 'perfect children', we are still a long way away from achieving this goal. Many 'desirable' characteristics such as height or intelligence are coded for by a **number** of genes. Often, we don't fully understand the interactions between them. In addition, **environmental factors** such as diet or education may be as important as the genes in producing these characteristics. So, at the present time, the potential for enhancing our children through genetic manipulation is decidedly limited.

Cloning – the ethical issues

In 1997, the birth of Dolly the sheep heralded the start of a new era in biotechnology. Mammalian cloning was possible. Since that day, scientists have raced to be the first to clone a human being. Those in authority, however, have not been so enthusiastic and cloning is banned in many countries. The *Human Reproductive Cloning Act 2001* made human reproductive cloning illegal in the UK.[6] The use of cloning procedures for other purposes, such as stem cell research, is only permitted under special government license.

What are the possible uses of cloning?
- Allowing infertile couples to have their own genetic children.

- Preventing carriers of X-linked or autosomal recessive disorders from passing on the conditions to their children.

- Preventing mitochondrially-inherited diseases.

- Obtaining stem cells to produce 'spare parts' such as organs for transplant.

The term 'cloning' can cover a variety of different techniques, including cloning embryos, cells or cell lines. Here we will focus mainly on the ethics of cloning for **reproductive** purposes.

No safe techniques for human reproductive cloning currently exist, despite the claims of a few maverick scientists. It is also illegal in the UK. Consequently, we realise that the ethics of cloning are of little practical importance to medical students or clinicians. Our discussion of the subject will be correspondingly brief.

The major arguments for and against reproductive cloning:

Argument in favour:

- People should be allowed to reproduce in the way they choose (i.e. we should respect their 'reproductive liberty').

- It would help infertile or gay couples to have children who are genetically their own.

- It could help prevent the transmission of certain genetic disorders.

Arguments against:

- Yuk!

- It involves killing embryos.

- It is playing God.

- It is racist and eugenic.

- It violates fundamental human rights – the right to an individual's genetic identity and the right to have two (biological) parents.

- It confuses family relationships and genealogy.

- It is unsafe. Dolly the sheep died prematurely, suffering from lung disease and arthritis, and cloned animals show a high rate of abnormality or disability per live birth.

As you can see, many of these arguments seem to be based more on gut instinct or emotional reaction than on valid reasoning. But is there any validity in the arguments themselves? We will briefly consider two common objections to cloning:

1. Cloning is a 'violation of fundamental human rights' as it violates each individual's 'right to his or her **own genetic identity**'. This argument was made by the European parliament.[7]

Firstly, does each individual have a right to his own genetic identity? By examining the case of twins, John Harris shows that a unique 'genetic identity' is not an essential part of personal identity, nor is it necessary for 'individuality'. If we are not disturbed by *'nature's clones'* (as Harris calls monozygotic twins) why should we feel so uncomfortable about artificially created clones?[4]

Secondly, does cloning violate human rights? Cloning occurs **naturally** at a rate of **1 in 270** pregnancies. In the case of monozygotic twins, does the mere existence of one twin threaten the human rights of the other? In the UK, over 200,000 monozygotic twin pregnancies will have occurred in our population of nearly 60 million people. Harris attacks this argument by saying 'If each of these is a violation of human rights, how are we to regard human rights violations on such a grand scale?' (p. 33)[4]

In addition, producing clones does not make copies of one *individual,* only of one particular **genotype.** Environmental factors also make a substantial contribution to the way a particular individual 'turns out'. For example, identical twins have the same genotype, but often very different personalities, likes and dislikes, and even appearances.

2. Cloning is **racist and eugenic:** if we clone certain individuals, it implies that we value their characteristics more highly than those of other individuals.

This is not really an argument about cloning itself, but about our reproductive choices in general. If this argument is to be used to ban cloning, we should also ban the following out of consistency: pre-natal and pre-implantation screening, egg and sperm donation, surrogacy, and even the choice of natural reproductive partner! All of them involve valuing certain characteristics over others.

Furthermore, as we argued in chapter 6, the fact that something can be misused does not necessarily justify banning it altogether. Safeguards can often be put in place to prevent or reduce abuse.

Summary

- The ethical issues in clinical genetics are similar to those in other areas of practice, but the **familial nature** of genetic information raises additional issues.

- Informed consent and adequate provision of information are vital before offering patients genetic testing.

- Genetic testing can have a variety of **benefits,** such as resolving uncertainty, allowing planning and enabling access to potential therapies.

- However, considerable social, psychological and financial **harms** can also result.

- Screening for adult onset conditions is rarely carried out in children.

- Gene therapy and cloning raise interesting ethical issues, but are not practically possible at the current time.

- Human cloning is currently **illegal** in the UK.

References

1. British Medical Association; Medical Ethics Today. London: BMJ Publishing Group, 2004.

2. Human Genome Project Information Website. URL: www.ornl.gov/sci/techresources/Human_Genome/home.shtml.

3. Committee on the Ethics of Gene Therapy. Report of the Committee on the Ethics of Gene Therapy. London: HMSO, 1992:21.

4. Harris J. *Clones, Genes and Immortality. Ethics and the Genetic Revolution.* Oxford: Oxford University Press, 1998.

5. Hope T, Savulescu J, Hendrick J. *Medical ethics and law: the core curriculum.* Edinburgh: Churchill Livingstone, 2003.

6. Human Reproductive Cloning Act 2001. URL: www.hmso.gov.uk/acts/acts2001/20010023.htm.

7. The European Parliament, Resolution on Cloning. 1997.

Children

Children are generally considered a vulnerable group in need of protection. Due to their young age, immaturity or inability to understand treatments, some children are unable to make autonomous decisions. At the same time, many of us feel that children should be empowered and that the wishes of older children should, at least in some cases, be respected. The law attempts to strike a balance between these two potentially conflicting attitudes.

Whatever their age and mental competence, all children have rights. Amongst others, they have a right to life, a right to freedom of expression, and a right not to be tortured, abused or neglected. The Convention on the Rights of Children, ratified by 192 countries, provides an extensive list of children's rights, although these are not legally enforceable. The Human Rights Act 1998, however, gives children certain enforceable rights. Article 3 of the Act, for example, protects *anyone* from inhuman or degrading treatment or punishment.

The law regarding children is, alas, quite confusing, and requires a few minutes' concentration.

Relevant law and ethics on the topic

- Children aged 16 or 17 are **assumed competent** and **can consent to treatment,** just like adults. Their consent to clinically indicated medical treatment should be respected **even if the parents disagree with the child's decision** (under the Family Law Reform Act 1969).

- If children aged 16 or 17 refuse treatment, however, their **refusal can be overridden if parents or doctors believe the refusal is not in the child's best interests.** Doctors can override a child's refusal if someone with parental authority gives consent. If a person with parental authority and the child refuse treatment, the doctor would need the permission of the courts to override the refusal.

The possibility of enforcing treatment is one of the major differences between minors and adults. Remember that competent adults can refuse any treatment, for whatever reason!

* Doctors should seek the views of all children – even young ones – and take those views into account when making decisions. This should help make a better evaluation of what constitutes the particular child's 'best interests'.

The reasoning behind the current law, which might seem illogical to many, is that the consequences of refusing life-saving treatment are so awful that this justifies overriding a child's autonomy. All the cases which come to the courts involve grave decisions which, if respected, may result in death or serious harm. The consequences of consenting to a treatment, however, are usually beneficial and so should be allowed.

True Story:
In 1999, Ms M, a 15 year-old girl who sustained acute heart failure, refused to have a heart transplant. She feared that she would lose her identity and be considered 'different'. The court gave consent to override her refusal.[1]

In balancing the risks and benefits, the benefits of denying her refusal (i.e. saving her life) were considered weightier than the risks of respecting her wish. In this case, the principle of beneficence trumped the principle of respect for autonomy!

Note that if she was 18 (and deemed competent), doctors would have had to respect her refusal.

---

* Children **under 16** can consent to treatment if they have the intelligence and understanding to know what is proposed (i.e. if they are 'Gillick' competent).

The Gillick case: Victoria Gillick, a devout Roman Catholic, appeared in court in the early 1980s to ask that none of her five daughters be offered birth control. All were under 16. Her appeal was ultimately rejected by the House of Lords. It was decided that a child under 16 requesting contraceptives could be given treatment without notifying the parents if the child had **'sufficient understanding and intelligence to enable him or her to *understand fully* what is proposed'.**[2] What was meant by 'understand fully' was left unclear.

Over the age of 16, people are **presumed competent** to make any decision, unless proved otherwise. For people **under 16, the opposite is true** – they are presumed incompetent unless proved otherwise.

- After the Gillick decision in the mid 1980s, it appeared that competent children could, by logical extension, also refuse treatment, but later cases suggested otherwise. In the case of R (1991), where a 15-year-old girl refused anti-psychotic treatment, the local authority made her a ward of court to obtain permission to provide anti-psychotic treatment. The Court of Appeal held that R was not competent to refuse treatment.

Assessing competence in children
To be deemed competent, children must show that they:

- Understand the options and their consequences.

- Can balance the pros and cons of each option and make a decision.

- Want to make a decision.

- Understand the reason and nature of the procedure.

- Understand the procedure's risks and side-effects.

- Are free from undue pressure.

Diagram summarizing the law on children's consent and refusal of treatment

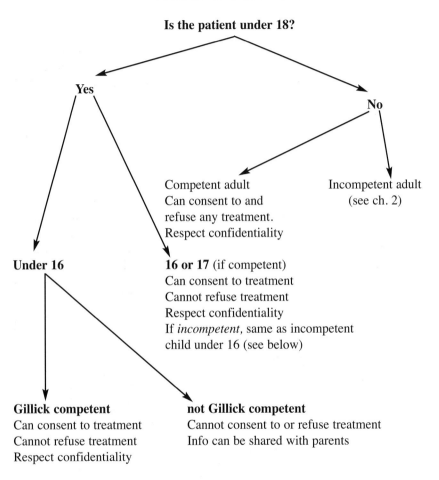

Is the patient under 18?

Yes

No

Competent adult
Can consent to and
refuse any treatment.
Respect confidentiality

Incompetent adult
(see ch. 2)

Under 16

16 or 17 (if competent)
Can consent to treatment
Cannot refuse treatment
Respect confidentiality
If *incompetent*, same as incompetent
child under 16 (see below)

Gillick competent
Can consent to treatment
Cannot refuse treatment
Respect confidentiality

not Gillick competent
Cannot consent to or refuse treatment
Info can be shared with parents

Parental responsibility for children

If the child is unable to consent, **the responsibility falls on the (birth) mother.** The
father is also responsible if:

1. He was married to the mother at the time of birth or conception, or

2. He is registered as the father on the child's birth certificate, even if he is not married to the mother (Adoption and Children Act 2002, s111).

If the father is not automatically responsible, the mother can still transfer responsibility to the father or other relatives, but she needs a legal document or court order to show this. Consent should be sought from **one holder of parental responsibility.** That person's decision should be respected unless the doctor thinks it is not in the best interests of the child. Remember that the doctor would need to obtain consent from the court to override the decision (except in a grave emergency, in which case the doctor should treat the child immediately).

In practice

If someone without parental responsibility (e.g. a school teacher) brings a child for treatment, the doctor should contact someone who does have the authority to consent on behalf of the child. If, however, this proves impossible and the child needs urgent treatment, the doctor should not put the child at risk by trying desperately to contact someone who can consent! He should act in the child's best interests (i.e. treat the kid).

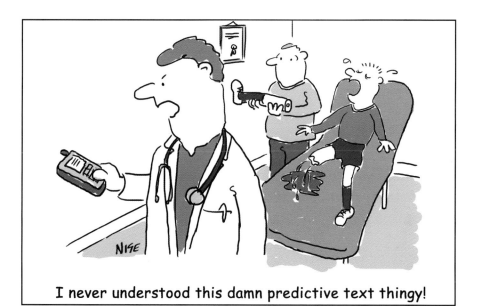

I never understood this damn predictive text thingy!

The court can consent on behalf of a child even if both the parents and the child refuse treatment. A familiar example is the case of Jehovah's Witnesses who decline blood transfusions for their sick children on religious grounds. The court can override, and have totally overridden, the parents' wishes. If they decline blood *for themselves,* however, the doctor should respect their refusal of treatment.

So, in the case of children, consent can come from:

1. a competent child

2. parents (or holders of parental responsibility)

3. the courts

As mentioned earlier, doctors can provide **life-saving treatment** in a **medical emergency,** even against the wishes of a child or the parents.

Common 'long essay' question with answer

Here is a typical essay question on this topic. We have provided a full answer, and incorporated new material in the essay. Don't be worried if you feel unable to produce a similar answer yourself! Medical students are not expected to provide such elaborate answers. Still, the essay is useful as an example of an excellent answer and as a means of conveying new information.

Note that, in this question, examiners are not looking for a 'correct' answer. However, this doesn't mean that any answer will do! There are still good and bad answers. What sets apart a piece of rubbish from a good answer is mainly the way your argument is backed up and developed.

'Is it morally justifiable to give minors the right to consent to treatment but not the right to refuse treatment?'

In the United Kingdom, adults may consent to or refuse treatment as long as they are deemed competent. An 18-year-old, for example, may refuse a life-saving blood transfusion for the most trivial of reasons – or indeed no reason at all – as long as he is competent. Children under 18, however, may consent to treatment if sufficiently competent but cannot refuse it if a person with parental authority or a court of law decide otherwise. Is this an ethical anomaly? If so, what is odd about it? On what grounds can it be criticised? Conversely, how can this position best be defended? The examination of the notion of 'consent' is the most obvious starting point in attempting to answer these questions.

If one consents to X, one willingly accepts that X be done. In the case of medical practice, the value of such consent is evident. It informs the doctor that the patient approves of the procedure, and provides a near-certain guarantee that he is acting in the patient's best interests. In modern medical ethics, where the principle of respect for autonomy predominates, respecting the patient's wishes is considered good in itself, falling within the category of 'best interests'. Obtaining a patient's consent also impacts on the potential success of a medical procedure, as the patient is more likely to take his pills or comply to a treatment regime if he supported the treatment in the first place. If hope plays a part in recovery, then a patient who consents to a treatment might hold greater hope in the treatment's success than one whose wishes were ignored and whose treatment was forcibly imposed. Finally, obtaining consent protects the doctor from charges of unlawful conduct (usually assault or battery).

Consent, then, is valuable for a number of ethical, clinical and legal reasons, but a more difficult question relates to the qualities required to give valid consent. One must be competent, but what is meant by 'competent'? What is clear is that the moral criteria for competence are not absolute, but vary according to the decision to be made. They are, in other words, decision-specific. A child can decide in which buttock to have his injection but can conceivably be too young to decide whether or not to have the injection. Even if the criteria are dependent on the particular decision, some basic requirements must be met. One must possess adequate cognitive abilities to balance the reasons for and against making a decision, which entails a knowledge of the risks and possible side-effects of the decision. No matter how competent, consent cannot be valid if the patient has received insufficient or biased information, or if he has failed to understand the doctor's disclosure. Finally, the patient's choice must be his own, free from coercion or undue pressure from the doctor or the patient's relatives.

How to assess the cognitive abilities of a person to determine his competence is subject to considerable debate, but this difficulty can be avoided in our discussion, as we are not trying to untangle the meaning of competence but rather its implications on issues relating to children's consent to and refusal of treatment. Assuming a child is competent, what other assumptions can be made?

For philosophers such as John Harris, one cannot *truly* consent to treatment if one is unable to refuse it.[3] If consent involves weighing up the pros and cons of treatment, then it must necessarily involve an awareness of the consequences of a refusal. Harris concludes 'So, to understand a proposed treatment well enough to consent to it is to understand the consequences of a refusal.' This seems logically correct. The impossibility of refusing treatment also makes consent meaningless, as it is no longer a genuine choice. For a choice to be real, there must be an achievable alternative. If the host at a dinner party asks a polite guest if he enjoyed the food he so painstakingly prepared, the guest's answer is fairly meaningless as the alternative – saying the food tasted like feet – is simply not an option. No realistic alternative means no free choice.

How can such a discrepancy be explained? One possible reason is that society feels an obligation to protect its more vulnerable members from a range of harms, and children, like the elderly or the mentally unfit, fall within the category of the 'vulnerable'. Besides, for society to function children must grow into healthy adults who will contribute to the work force and inject resources into the system. But the question then is 'are competent children more vulnerable than competent adults?'. If the level of competence is identical, then vulnerability – i.e. the ability to be coerced or exploited – cannot be higher in one than in the other. One could argue that physical weakness can contribute to vulnerability but, even if we accept this, it would apply only to a certain group of children. Many 15 year-old children are physically stronger than the average adult.

Another possible explanation to account for the discrepancy is the authority of a qualified professional. By consenting to a treatment, one is following the recommendations of a highly-trained expert. By refusing a treatment, however, one is willingly going against the advice of an expert. For this very reason, consent and refusal are not treated identically; the latter requires much stronger justification.

To use the language of principlism, the law is overriding the principle of respect for the child's autonomy with the principle of beneficence. As stipulated in the Children

Act, practitioners should do what is best for the child and, in cases where respecting a child's decision could lead to serious harm, this could justify imposing treatment on the child. But a similar question to the previous case on vulnerability arises: why should this weighing of principles apply to children and not to adults? Why is it in the best interests of the *child* (not society as a whole) to stay alive against his will and not in the best interests of an adult? Does what constitutes our 'best interests' shift with our advancing age? Both the argument from vulnerability and the argument from best interests prompt the following question: what is it that adults have that children don't? Is it rationality, maturity, wisdom, self-awareness, intelligence or some other characteristic? Is it a combination of these?

A common critique of the age cut-off is the arbitrariness of the cut-off point. Is a child sufficiently mature to buy a packet of cigarettes or a national lottery ticket at age 16, but not so the day before his 16th birthday? No one would believe this to be true, but that is not to say that cut-off points are unnecessary. Indeed, almost all cut-off points can be considered arbitrary. The problem, in our case, stems from the conflict between the continuity of cognitive faculties and the bipolar nature of rights. One can be more or less competent to consent to X, but one cannot have more or less of a legal right to Y (e.g. vote, drive, etc.) This leads to apparent incongruencies in the areas immediately to the sides of the cut-off point. What proponents of the critique would claim is that one cannot correlate competence with age, and that cut-off points based on age should therefore be removed. A counter to this would be to acknowledge the fallibility of the correlation, but to add that this is the least fallible of the alternatives, as well as the most practicable. Generally speaking, a 10-year-old is less competent to make an important medical decision than a 30-year-old.

Another argument in favour of allowing competent children to refuse treatment can be called the argument from inconsistency. Society wishes to protect its children but, at the same time, strives to empower them and give them responsibilities. The principle of *doli incapax,* which established that children between 10 and 13 were incapable of moral responsibility for a crime, was abolished in 1998. Today, a child as young as 10 in England and Wales can be held responsible for a crime he has committed. In other European countries, the age of criminal responsibility varies from 12 (Greece, Holland) to 18 (Belgium, Luxembourg). The inconsistency is apparent: a 10-year-old may be assumed sufficiently competent to commit a crime and to understand the right or wrong of his action, but a 17-year-old cannot refuse medical treatment. On April 3, 2003, Scott Hain was executed in Oklahoma for a crime he committed when he was 17. The previous year, three minors were executed in Texas. Closer to home, the two boys who murdered Jamie Bulger in 1993 were tried as adults in court, even though they were only 11 at the time of the trial.

From a purely logical viewpoint, allowing a competent child to consent to treatment without allowing him to refuse is indefensible. If X is as competent as Y to refuse an operation, then both should be either allowed to consent or refuse. Consistency is the key word. As we have seen, the inconsistency is difficult to justify if we adopt the perspective of the individual in question, although it is easier if we adopt the broader perspective of society as a whole, whose policy makers are faced with the unenviable task of balancing the rights of the individual with the need to protect vulnerable groups.

Although logically imperfect and, indeed, unfortunate for those children competent enough to refuse treatment, my own view is that there is little evidence that a better alternative exists. So called 'child liberationists' often list the inconsistencies in the law without suggesting realistic ways to remedy the situation. Many 'child protectionists', on the other hand, are aware that certain children are sufficiently capable to make complex medical choices, but believe any change in law will cause more harm than good. There is therefore a common ground between the two parties: both agree that some children are as competent as adults. The difference lies in the practical entailment of this simple observation. Our efforts should therefore focus on ways to best incorporate this ethical anomaly into healthcare policy and medical law.

Child abuse

- Doctors have a **duty to protect children** from physical, sexual, and emotional abuse, including neglect.

- The doctor's **primary responsibility is to the child,** not the child's family. For this reason, the doctor may share relevant information about suspected abuse with other members of the healthcare team without parental consent.

- If a doctor suspects child abuse (through suspicious findings during examination, the child's own account, or a member of the public) he should **contact social services or the police promptly.** The doctor should note the referral in the child's health records.

If the situation is considered sufficiently serious, the relevant authority may temporarily remove the child from the parents.

- For incompetent children, doctors should act in the **child's best interests.** This may include breaching confidentiality to alert the relevant authorities.

• When dealing with competent children who may have been abused, doctors should discuss the possibility of alerting the authorities with the child. If the child refuses, the doctor should act in the child's best interests. The doctor should also consider whether, and how, his actions will affect others, including the child's siblings. The doctor should balance the harms and benefits of breaching confidentiality with those of non-disclosure.

• If the local authority asks for assistance in investigating cases of child abuse, doctors should **cooperate if they believe this will prevent serious harm to the child.**

• If appropriate, doctors should involve the parents in the situation. They should inform the parents that a relevant authority has been contacted to resolve the problem. Nevertheless, there may be cases (such as those involving sexual abuse) when alerting the parents is not recommended as this might aggravate the situation and pose further risks to the child.

Summary

• Children who are **16 or 17 can consent** to treatment (if competent) but **cannot refuse** treatment if doctors believe this is not in the child's best interests.

• Children under 16 can consent to treatment if **Gillick competent** (but cannot refuse treatment).

• In the case of children, consent can come from a **competent child,** a **parent** or **holder of parental responsibility,** or the **courts.**

• Doctors should **always act in the best interests of the child.** This may involve breaching confidentiality.

• Doctors should **alert the relevant authorities** if they suspect a child has been abused.

References

1. Re M 2 FLR 1097, 1999.

2. Gillick v. W. Norfolk AHA 3 All ER 402, 1985.

3. Harris J. Consent and end of life decisions. *Journal of Medical Ethics* 2003 29:10-15.

The sad, the mad and the bad: mental disorders and disabilities

In chapter 2, we saw how the principle of respect for patient autonomy requires doctors to obtain informed consent before treating any competent patient. However, we only glanced over the treatment of patients suffering from mental disorders. The majority of such patients are treated as voluntary or 'informal' patients. That is, they are treated with their consent, and the ethical issues surrounding their care are no different to those of other patients.

However, some mentally disordered patients can **lose insight** into their illness or their need for treatment. These patients may need to be detained under the **Mental Health Act (1983).** This is an interesting area in medical ethics, as it is the only situation in which doctors can treat competent patients *without* their consent. Such treatment is governed by **strict legal requirements** in the form of the Mental Health Act.

Medical students should know the basics of the law regarding the treatment of mentally disordered patients. This chapter provides an introduction to the relevant law and ethics on mental disorders.

What is a 'mental disorder'?

Doctors can only legally detain a patient under the Mental Health Act (MHA) if they are **suffering from a mental disorder.** Therefore, it is important to clarify the meaning of the term 'mental disorder'. Rather confusingly, the meaning of the term depends on the section of the Mental Health Act used to detain a patient. Fortunately, you only need to know two main sections of the MHA: **Sections 2 and 3.**

A 'Section 3' is used to detain someone with a *known* mental disorder in hospital in order to **provide treatment** for that disorder. To admit a patient for treatment under section 3, they must be suffering from one of **4 specified categories** of mental disorder:

1. **Mental Illness:**
   This term is not defined further in the Act. Clinical judgement is used to decide what is included (see later discussion).

2. **Mental Impairment:**
   A **developmental** abnormality that causes **significant impairment of intelligence and social functioning** (i.e. patients with *learning disability*), and is associated with **abnormally aggressive or seriously irresponsible conduct.**

3. **Severe Mental Impairment:**
   As mental impairment, but more severe.

4. **Psychopathic Disorder:**
   A **persistent disorder** or **disability of mind** (with or without significant impairment of intelligence) which results in **abnormally aggressive or seriously irresponsible conduct.**

NOTE: The term 'psychopathic disorder' is used here as a *legal term*. It can apply to **any personality disorder which causes behavioural problems** (not just 'psychopathic' or 'dissocial' personality disorder).

A '**Section 2**' is invoked to admit a patient to hospital for the **diagnosis** of a suspected mental disorder. As the diagnosis may be unclear at this stage, the term 'mental disorder' does not refer to any specific categories of disorder, as required for admission under section 3.

But you cannot detain ....

In the past, doctors have detained sexually promiscuous patients on mental health grounds. Nowadays, the Mental Health Act specifically states that the following reasons are **NOT** *in themselves sufficient* to detain people:

• Dependence on drugs and alcohol

• Promiscuity

• Sexual deviancy

Point of debate: what is meant by the term 'mental illness'?
Some medical ethicists and civil liberties campaigners have commented on the definitional vagueness of the term 'mental illness' in the Mental Health Act. This lack of definition may seem odd, especially as most patients admitted to hospital under the Act are detained under this category.

A Department of Health consultation document, published alongside the 1983 Act, described 'mental illness' as:

> **an illness including delusional beliefs, abnormal perceptions and disordered thinking.**[1]

This is what most psychiatrists would call psychosis.
In practice, it is not just psychotic illnesses (e.g. schizophrenia) that are treated under the MHA. For example, a severely depressed, suicidal patient may require treatment under the MHA for their depression. The final decision about which 'mental illnesses' need treatment under the MHA requires a common-sense approach from doctors. It would be rare to detain someone for a morbid fear of socks, no matter how disabling!

What conditions are necessary for use of the MHA?

Before detaining someone under the MHA, several important conditions must be met:

1. They must be suffering from a mental disorder of a type and severity that makes **treatment in hospital appropriate** (i.e. you cannot provide suitable treatment at home or in a community care facility).

2. Detention is in **the interests of the patient's health and safety,** or of **other people's health and safety.**

3. A third condition applies only to those with **personality disorders.** For detention to be legal, treatment must be likely to **improve their condition,** or **prevent it from getting worse.** In practice, many psychiatrists are reluctant to keep certain patients with personality disorders in hospital as they feel that these conditions are not readily treatable.

The patient should first be offered to be **admitted informally** to hospital. If the patient declines the offer, doctors can then consider using the compulsory powers of the Mental Health Act.

Who can section a patient under the MHA?

If you are considering becoming a psychiatrist to lock up your annoying younger brother, think again. The requirements for sectioning a patient are quite strict. **Two doctors and an Approved Social Worker** should agree that the patient should be sectioned (except in an emergency, where the conditions are less stringent). One of the doctors is usually a consultant or registrar in psychiatry and the other is often the patient's GP.

The patient's nearest relative can object to the patient's admission to hospital. However, if this objection is felt to be unreasonable, the Approved Social Worker can apply to the County Court to 'displace' the nearest relative. This allows doctors to go ahead with treatment in the patient's best interests.

The patient's right to appeal

The patient is informed of his right to appeal on admission. Indeed, many units encourage patients to appeal so that they understand that their detention is not unjust. Patients are offered free legal representation at each stage of the appeal process.

A patient admitted under section 2 (or their representative) can make this appeal at any time **in the first two weeks** after admission. Patients detained under section 3 are entitled to **one hearing in the first 6 months** of treatment, **one in the second 6 months,** and **one per year thereafter.**

The appeal process has two stages. It goes first to the **managers of the hospital** in which the patient is detained. The managers appoint a panel of lay persons, who undergo training in the Mental Health Act. On most occasions, patients are not discharged by this panel, and the appeal progresses to a **Mental Health Review Tribunal.** The Tribunal is made up of a lawyer, an independent psychiatrist and a lay person. The consultant in charge of the patient's care presents reasons why he should not be discharged. A solicitor represents the patient's view.

Implications of the Mental Health Act

The Mental Health Act is arguably a unique piece of legislation, as it can deprive a person of their liberty indefinitely. Once detained, patients can be **treated against their will.** As we saw in chapter 2, this would **constitute an assault under normal circumstances.** The concepts of consent and capacity, which are so dear to us in the rest of medical practice, are not given much weight in the current mental health legalisation. There is a huge chasm between the ethics of treating patients under the Mental Health Act and the ethics of treating patients in the rest of medical practice.

Why is specific mental health legislation needed?

It could be argued that specific Mental Health legislation is not needed at all. What is wrong with treating the mentally ill in the same way as the physically ill? If a mentally ill patient who needed treatment was deemed incompetent, why could we not act in their best interests and treat them under common law? Let us consider arguments to justify the existence of specific Mental Health legislation.

Arguments in favour of specialist Mental Health Law:
1. **A more paternalistic approach is justified in the case of mental disorder.**
   A mental illness can profoundly affect the ability of sufferers to function normally.

> **Example:** Many patients with schizophrenia have **no insight** into their illness. They do not believe that they are ill. They are terrorised by auditory hallucinations. You try to explain to them that these voices are not those of real people, that they are inside their head, and occur as a result of their illness. Yet they continue to believe that the voices are real and live in constant fear.

Anyone who has worked on a psychiatric ward will know how distressing this can be for the patient, their family and the staff looking after them. Many mentally ill patients cannot make decisions about their treatment, or about other aspects of their life.

> **Example:** Patients with bi-polar disorder may get into considerable trouble during a manic episode. They can run up thousands of pounds of debt in a single weekend. Some female patients may become sexually disinhibited and have unprotected sex with several partners. Once the manic episode ends, they are left to live with the consequences of their actions.

The main purpose of the Mental Health Act is to help those people who may be **too unwell to make appropriate decisions about hospitalisation, treatment or management of their property.**[2]

This is clearly a more paternalistic approach than that used with other patients. Can we justify this difference? First, consider why paternalism is usually thought to be a bad thing. One reason is that it **violates people's autonomy.** In the case of serious mental illness, however, people's autonomy is often (although not always) significantly reduced.

As well as recognising the patient's need for liberty, there is also **a need to uphold his right to treatment,** even if the patient himself may not realise that he needs it. However, things become ethically tricky when a patient's autonomy is not diminished, and they are competent *despite* the presence of the mental disorder. This will be discussed shortly, when we consider whether this more paternalistic approach discriminates against the mentally ill.

2. **The time frame of treatment calls for special legislation.**
   The use of common law to treat patients in their best interests is usually employed in emergency situations. Patients either recover (and regain capacity), or do not, within a few days or weeks.

   On the other hand, most mental disorders are chronic and require long term treatment. It is therefore important to make sure that powers are in place **to prevent misuse** of the Act.

3. **Mental illness can affect capacity in other ways.**[3]
   A third argument revolves around the *true competence* of mentally disordered patients to make autonomous choices about their own lives. They may be deemed 'competent' by the normal process of assessing competence, but is this assessment sufficient in the case of mental illness?

> Consider the case of a severely depressed adult refusing antidepressant medication. The reason for his refusal is that he considers himself worthless and feels that he does not deserve to live.

How do we decide whether this patient is competent? As we explained in chapter 2, the usual procedure for assessing capacity requires us to ask the question: 'is the patient able to **retain information** long enough to **process** it, to **understand** it and to **use** it make a reasoned decision?'.

When answering the question, we consider whether any **cognitive impairment** is affecting his ability to understand, process and reason. If the patient suffers from dementia, his inability to achieve these key tasks may be obvious. In psychiatry, doctors commonly consider **additional factors** (other than cognitive ability) in their assessment of capacity. A leading psychiatry textbook stresses the need to identify these other factors, as they may *interfere with capacity*. They include:

• **delusions**

• **hallucinations**

• **altered values** in affective disorders such as depression and mania

• **lack of emotional maturity**[4]

In the case of the depressed patient, it can be argued that *altered values* are impacting upon his capacity. His sense of worthlessness and dejection is probably not a truly held, autonomous belief, but a product of his depressive illness. Respecting his autonomy, some might argue, is to **respect what he would have wanted if not depressed.** This can be difficult to determine. He may have become depressed *because* of his existential angst. The depression may have been caused by his true, autonomous beliefs! However, we can assume that most people, when not depressed, would rather live than die.

At the current time, this idea of other factors affecting on capacity is not built into the current mental health legislation. So legally, you can override this patient's refusal of treatment as he is **suffering from a mental illness** and the treatment is **in the interests of his own health.** You do not specifically have to consider the issue of competence.

Ethically, however the presence of altered values resulting from the depression is probably the strongest argument for overriding the patient's wishes.[3] Nevertheless, it is difficult to demonstrate that his current values do not represent his real values.

A second function of the Mental Health Act is to provide for people with mental disorders who are **charged with, or convicted of, an offence.** The ethical issues relating to this are discussed further below.

Does the MHA discriminate against the mentally ill?

Some authors have suggested that mental health legislation discriminates against mentally ill patients.[3] There are two main areas of controversy:

* Firstly, under the MHA, **doctors can override a refusal of treatment by a competent patient with a mental disorder.** The treatment of patients under the MHA is thus inconsistent with that of any other patient under common law. In normal circumstances, a patient is free to refuse treatment whatever the consequences to his health. Failing to respect the refusal of treatment is a legal offence. However, a mentally ill patient can be competent (under the current definitions we use) and still be treated against his will.

* The second concern relates to the use of the Act for the **protection of others.** Mentally disordered patients can potentially be **detained for an indefinite period** if deemed a danger to society, even if they have committed no crime. There is no mechanism under criminal law to imprison those who have not been convicted of a crime, however dangerous we may judge them to be.

Are these purely theoretical concerns or do they impact significantly on the practice of caring for mentally ill patients?

In reality, it is uncommon for doctors to forcibly override a competent but mentally ill patient's refusal of treatment. The majority of patients are 'informal' and even those initially reluctant to come into hospital usually accept the need for treatment once admitted. Only rarely do doctors have to give treatments against a patient's will. When this is required, however, the experience may be distressing for both patient and staff.

It can be argued that the short-term distress of compulsory medication needs to be balanced against the long-term benefits of treatment. Despite this, many ethicists still lament the fact that the requirements for consent are so different for mentally ill patients than for others. The new mental health legislation currently in draft is likely to include *some recognition of capacity* in the treatment of patients who refuse medical care.

The issue of detaining mentally disordered patients for the **protection of others** is even more contentious. At the present time, only a small number of patients are detained in this way. However, the 2002 draft of the new Mental Health legislation planned new laws for dangerous patients suffering from dissocial (psychopathic) personality disorder. This issue is the subject of much debate.

The government's plan was to remove the 'treatability' criterion of the 1983 Act, allowing the detention of patients suffering from 'dangerous severe personality disorder' **before any crime is committed.** Many psychiatrists are reluctant to admit such patients under the MHA, due to the difficulty of treating the condition. The profession therefore spoke out strongly against this move. The BMA called it 'threatening civil liberties and potentially turning therapeutic legislation into a vehicle for social control' (p. 128).[5]

For mentally ill patients considered dangerous to others, a balance must be found between 1) **maintaining the therapeutic environment** for patients and 2) **protecting public safety.** Ideally, this should involve using the least restrictive treatment compatible with public safety, but debate continues about how restrictive this should be.

What is the future for mental health legislation?

Mental health legislation in England and Wales is currently under review. Some of the problems with the existing Mental Health Act are likely to be addressed in the new bill mentioned earlier. In 1995, the Law Commission described the MHA as 'unsystematic and full of glaring gaps', saying in addition that it had 'failed to keep up with developments in our understanding of the rights and needs of those with mental disability'.[6]

In particular, the MHA does not reflect the growing shift away from inpatient hospital treatment to community-based care. Under the current Act, there is no framework to ensure that patients take their medication whilst out of hospital. This leads to a vicious cycle of 'revolving door admissions'. Patients who refuse their medication relapse and eventually have to be admitted to hospital against their will, thus damaging the therapeutic relationship.

As previously mentioned, a draft bill to replace the MHA was published in 2002. After strong criticisms from mental health staff, patients and their families, however, the bill has been delayed for substantial redrafting.[7] In Scotland, legislation was updated in 2003.[8] The new Act emphasises an ethical approach to treatment and sets out a number of principles, including:

- **Non-discrimination,** as far as possible, compared to the processes used to treat patients without mental disorders.

- **Informal** care wherever possible, with minimal use of compulsory treatment.

- **Least restrictive treatment** – treatment provided in the manner least restrictive to patients that is compatible with the safety of others.

The principles above seem to correspond pretty closely to what psychiatrists strive to achieve in practice. Whatever the frameworks used to justify treatment decisions in the new English and Welsh legislation, the situation on the ground may remain much as it is now.

Treating patients under the MHA – seeking consent

While treating a patient under the Mental Health Act, doctors should still **obtain consent** in the normal way, before undertaking any examination or treatment. Establishing a collaborative and trusting relationship with the patient is particularly important when working with patients detained under the Mental Health Act. Many of them are anxious or suspicious as a result of their illness and may be very vulnerable. A diagnosis of mental illness can still be very stigmatising for both patients and families, and they may need considerable support to come to terms with it. A successful therapeutic relationship with staff is often an important step to recovery, but this can be put under great strain if compulsory treatment is required. Thus, the non-consensual administration of medications or other treatment under the MHA is **used only as a last resort.**

What treatments fall under the scope of the Mental Health Act?

In exceptional circumstances, admission under section 3 of the MHA allows some necessary treatments to be given against the wishes of the patient. However, there are important restrictions on the treatment that can be given:

- A patient can only be treated for the **mental disorder** for which he has been detained.

- He *cannot* be treated without his consent for a **physical disorder** unless that is the **cause of,** or **directly related to,** the mental disorder.

- The use of **drug treatments** for longer than **3 months,** or the use of **electroconvulsive therapy (ECT)** can only be carried out with either consent from the patient or a favourable second opinion from an independent doctor.

- For some more drastic treatment options, **patient consent** is still required. These include **psychosurgery** and the **implantation of hormones** to reduce male sex drive. Both patient consent *and* a second opinion are required in such cases.

Medical ethicists have long been interested in which medical conditions fall under the Mental Health Act. The famous case of Mr C illustrates this area of controversy:

> **The case of Re C[9]**
> Mr C was a 68-year-old paranoid schizophrenic. He suffered from grandiose delusions that he was a famous doctor. In 1993, he developed gangrene in his foot while detained in a secure hospital.
>
> He was taken to a general hospital, where a consultant surgeon told him he had an 85% chance of death if his leg was not amputated below the knee. He refused the amputation, confident that he would survive with the help of God and the medical staff. However, he did acknowledge the possibility of death if he kept the leg, saying he would *"rather die with two feet than live with one."*
>
> This case went to the High Court which ruled that although C's schizophrenia did impact on his general capacity, he was **competent to refuse the amputation.** He had understood and retained the relevant information, in his own way believed it, and had therefore arrived at a choice. The hospital was not allowed to amputate without his express written consent, either now or in the future if his mental capacity deteriorated further. Mr C survived without the amputation.

Mr C's capacity to refuse treatment for the gangrenous foot was assessed on the basis of *cognitive abilities only.* The fact that Mr C's grandiose delusions (that he was a world-famous surgeon) might have affected the decision was irrelevant since his cognitive reasoning was intact. To some, this may seem illogical. However, this case illustrates an important principle: the assessment of capacity for the *physical* disorders of patients detained under the MHA is the **same as that of any other patient.**

Summary

- Mentally disordered patients can be detained under the Mental Health Act (1983) if this is in the **interests of the patient's health or safety, or the health and safety of others.**

- Hospital treatment is only considered if community treatment is not sufficient. **Informal admission** should be offered first.

- Patients have the **right to appeal** against their detention and are offered free legal representation.

- Currently there is **no recognition of the concept of capacity** in mental health legislation. This can be said to discriminate against the mentally ill as competent patients suffering from a mental illness can be treated against their will.

- Ethical issues also arise from the use of the MHA to detain a patient for the protection of others.

- You must still **seek consent** from patients who are detained under the MHA. Compulsory treatment is used only as a last resort.

- **Restrictions apply** to treatment under the MHA. A second opinion is needed for the use of drug treatments lasting more than 3 months and the use of ECT.

- **Unrelated physical disorders cannot be compulsorily treated under the MHA.**

- Mental Health legislation is currently under review.

References

1. *Department of Health and Welsh Office Mental Health Act 1983; Code of Practice*. London: Stationary Office, 1999.

2. Doolan B. An introduction to law relevant to mentally disordered offenders. *Criminal Behaviour and Mental Health* 2004;14:S12-S18.

3. Hope T, Savulescu J, Hendrick J. *Medical ethics and law: the core curriculum*. Edinburgh: Churchill Livingstone, 2003.

4. Gelder M, Mayou R, Cowen P. *Shorter Oxford Textbook of Psychiatry*. Fourth ed. Oxford: Oxford University Press, 2001.

5. British Medical Association; Medical Ethics Today. London: BMJ Publishing Group, 2004.

6. Law Commission. *Mental incapacity*. London: HMSO, 1995:2.

7. Department of Health Draft Mental Health Bill, 2002.

8. Mental Health (Care and Treatment) Act (Scotland) s1, 2003.

9. Re C (adult: refusal of medical treatment) 1 All ER 819, 1994.

Questions of life and death: life, death, dying and killing

In this chapter, we will focus on the legal and ethical aspects of end-of-life care, the definition and logistics of 'Do Not Resuscitate' orders, and the certification of death. The chapter closes with a brief overview of key issues in organ transplantation.

Euthanasia and physician assisted suicide

Few debates in medical ethics generate as much controversy and disagreement as euthanasia.

Euthanasia can be defined as **'the intentional killing of a patient by act or omission as part of their medical treatment'.**[1]

There are several kinds of euthanasia:

• Active
• Passive
• Voluntary
• Non-voluntary
• Involuntary

What is the difference between the various types of euthanasia?

Active euthanasia

An active step is taken to intentionally end the patient's life (e.g. giving a lethal drug). There are three types of active euthanasia: voluntary, non-voluntary, and involuntary. They are **all illegal** in England. The difference between them relates to *consent*.

- **Voluntary active euthanasia** – An active step is taken to end the life of a competent person **with their consent**. In most cases, the person is suffering from a progressive terminal illness, such as motor neurone disease, and has asked to be euthanised. Voluntary active euthanasia is the only type of active euthanasia that is lawful in some countries, and is generally the type of active euthanasia referred to in end-of-life debates.

- **Non-voluntary active euthanasia** – An active step is taken to end the life of an **incompetent person**. The patient is unable to request euthanasia. An example would be a severely disabled baby.

- **Involuntary active euthanasia** – An active step is taken to end the life of a competent person **against their wishes.**

> **In brief:**
> Voluntary = with patient consent
> Non-voluntary = no patient consent
> Involuntary = against patient's wishes

Passive euthanasia

This is when death is intentionally brought about by **omitting to provide treatment.** Examples include the decision to withhold or withdraw life-prolonging treatment, or not to administer antibiotics so that a patient succumbs to an infection.

The difference between active and passive euthanasia is summed up in the 'killing and letting die' debate (see below). Active euthanasia is seen as killing, whereas passive euthanasia is seen as letting die. The BMA states that 'withdrawing or withholding treatment differs fundamentally from intentionally ending life'(p. 389).[1]

- In certain circumstances, **passive euthanasia may be lawful** in England although it is not usually called 'euthanasia'..

- **All forms** of **active** euthanasia are **illegal.**

Physician assisted suicide (PAS) differs from euthanasia in that it is **the patient himself,** not the doctor, who takes the **final step** to end his life. The doctor may or may not be present at the time of death, but he will have helped the patient end his life. This help could take a number of forms, from providing lethal drugs to giving advice on how the person could end his life. **PAS, like all cases of assisting suicide, is illegal in the UK.**

Summary of the law on end-of-life medicine

The law states that :

- Active euthanasia is illegal.

- Assisting suicide is a criminal offence (maximum sentence: 14 years in prison).

- Passive euthanasia is not necessarily illegal.

The real cases below illustrate the legal position on euthanasia and assisted suicide:

Case 1 – Active euthanasia

Lillian Boyes, a 70-year-old woman, suffered from rheumatoid arthritis which could no longer be controlled by analgesics. She repeatedly asked her rheumatologist, Dr Cox, to help her die. He injected her with a lethal dose of potassium chloride. As there was some doubt over the exact cause of death, Dr Cox was found guilty of attempted murder, rather than the **usual charge of murder.**

Case 2 – Assisted suicide

Diane Pretty suffered from motor neurone disease and repeatedly expressed a desire to have her husband assist her suicide. Mrs Pretty was not distressed by her current pain, but by the prospect of her impending suffering and loss of dignity. She sought an undertaking from the Director of Public Prosecutions that her husband would not be prosecuted under the 1961 Suicide Act if he helped her die. She lost the case in the Domestic Courts, but took it to the European Court of Human Rights. There she argued her case on several points in the European Convention of Human Rights, including:

- Article 2: the right to life (and therefore, she argued, the right to choose when to die)

- Article 3: the right to be free from inhuman or degrading treatment (which she believed further medical intervention would entail)

- Article 8: protection of private life (Mrs Pretty said the state was unduly interfering in her right to choose to die)

• Article 14: the right to be free from discrimination (here she argued that if able-bodied people are allowed to commit suicide, it is discriminatory not to afford the same right, with the extra help needed, to disabled people)

The European Court of Human Rights unanimously rejected her request. A transcript of the Court's judgement is available online: http://www.genethique.org/en/folders/dossiers/euthanasia/case_pretty.htm

Case 3 – Passive euthanasia
Tony Bland was a 21-year-old left in a permanent vegetative state (PVS) after the Hillsborough football stadium disaster in 1989. In 1993, the courts decided that artificial hydration and nutrition could be withdrawn, even though this would inevitably lead to his death. Hydration and nutrition were classed as 'treatments', rather than basic care, and so could be withdrawn as futile. The judges were of the opinion that, since Tony Bland had no interests at all, withholding treatment did not go against his best interests.

The law does not make a distinction between withdrawing and withholding treatment. For example, the law considers removing artificial ventilation to be passive, rather than active treatment. Legally, it is equivalent to not providing treatment (all other things being equal).

This has important practical consequences. If it were illegal for doctors to withdraw treatment once it started, it could be argued that doctors might be reluctant to start treating at all. This all-or-nothing situation would have bad consequences for doctors and patients. Under the current system, doctors can begin treating patients who have a small chance of recovery safe in the knowledge that they can stop the treatment if no progress is made.

How to avoid assisting the suicide of patients

It is not unusual for patients to express a wish to die. This may put doctors in a difficult position. To minimize the risk of spending time in jail for assisting the suicide of a patient, the BMA recommends that doctors should not:

• Advise patients on how to kill themselves (e.g. by specifying a lethal quantity of paracetamol tablets.)

- Intentionally prescribe or supply drugs to allow patients to shorten their lives.

- Provide any information (e.g. leaflets, names of 'sympathetic' colleagues) that will allow patients to shorten their lives.

> **An anonymous GP:**
> *"If someone asked me to help them commit suicide, I would (probably – depending on the reason) try to dissuade them from that course of action, and recommend some sort of sympathetic guidance service (like the 'Samaritans'). I would not give any further advice on how to succeed in the suicide attempt."*

As the laws on euthanasia and PAS differ from country to country, some claim that this will lead to '**suicide tourism**' with people travelling to these countries to be killed or to be allowed to die. Reginald Crew, a 74-year-old sufferer of motor neurone disease, travelled to Switzerland in 2002 with the company Dignitas, for PAS. In England, family members who knowingly help such persons plan their 'suicide' trip can be charged with assisting a suicide.

Should voluntary active euthanasia be legalised?

There is a considerable degree of public support for the legalisation of voluntary active euthanasia. Some common reasons in support of this position include:

- The **law is inconsistent.** If suicide is not illegal, then why shouldn't voluntary active euthanasia also be permitted? Some claim that this apparent inconsistency discriminates against disabled people who are unable to kill themselves.

- Withdrawing and withholding life-prolonging treatment (passive euthanasia) is already practised. Often, **a faster death** would cause **less distress** for the patient and their family. Large doses of opiates are often given to terminally ill people in the knowledge that they will hasten death, as well as relieve pain. Would it not be more honest and open to give treatments purely to shorten life without invoking the dubious doctrine of 'double effect'? (How the doctrine of double effect applies to passive euthanasia is explained below.)

- Respect for **autonomy**. Respect for autonomy should allow a competent person to control not only his life but also his death, and should **include respecting someone's genuine wish to die.** After all, we allow competent adults to refuse any medical treatment, even if this entails their certain death. We saw in chapter 2 that people differ in their interpretation of what is in their best interests. The concept of 'best interests' has an important subjective component. Mr Smith may find his severe illness tolerable but Mr Jones, who suffers from the same condition with the same degree of severity, may find it unbearable. Mr Smith may want to live for as long as he possibly can, despite the considerable discomfort, whereas Mr Jones may want to die immediately. The principle of respect for autonomy arguably requires us to respect the wishes of both Mr Smith and Mr Jones, so long as they have good reasons to justify their decision.

There are also strong arguments against voluntary active euthanasia:

- **Palliative care** is so effective that active euthanasia is unnecessary. Some also fear that the legalisation of euthanasia will divert funding away from palliative care services.

- The '**slippery slope**' argument. This argument claims that the legalisation of voluntary active euthanasia would mark the beginning of an **undesirable slide** to the killing of people who may not really wish to die, such as those who consider themselves a burden on their families or on society. Note that this is an empirical form of the slippery slope (see chapter 6 for details).

Another slippery slope argument is that, even with initially strict guidelines on who could request euthanasia, the conditions may become **less stringent** once it is legalised. People who at present would not be considered for euthanasia might be able to obtain it in the future.

Dr Andrew Fergusson, who in 1991 became chairman of HOPE (Healthcare Opposed to Euthanasia) believes that the *option* to choose euthanasia might gradually become an *obligation* to be euthanised. Elderly persons, through a combination of altruism and societal pressure, may feel obliged to 'opt' for euthanasia. (p. 55)[2]

- Legalising euthanasia would **change the role of doctors**. Some argue that euthanasia goes against the fundamental aim of medicine, which is to improve people's health and preserve life. This argument rests on *one interpretation* of the aims of medicine. If we accept that part of the aim is to alleviate suffering, however, euthanasia may not be contrary to the aims of medicine.

The **public perception of doctors** could also be irreparably damaged by legalising euthanasia. If doctors were required to end life as well as to save it, the public might view doctors in a different light and lose confidence in the medical profession. **Doctors might no longer be seen as healers, but also as executioners.** These multiple roles of the doctor might impact upon the doctor-patient relationship.

More moral arguments in the euthanasia debate

Double effect

The doctrine of double effect was discussed in some detail in chapter 6. In brief, it encapsulates the idea that there is a moral difference between intending an outcome and foreseeing an outcome. A doctor may be allowed to prescribe pain-relieving drugs which he intends for pain-relief, even though he forsees that such a dose might shorten the patient's life. However, according to the doctrine, no doctor is allowed to prescribe drugs with the **intention** of shortening the patient's life.

As we mentioned in chapter 6, the doctrine of double-effect is criticised on several grounds. Speaking about the doctrine of double effect, Lord Walton of Detchant argued that 'if Dr Cox, the rheumatologist, had given his patient massive doses of a sedative such as diazepam or one of its derivatives, so that the patient had gone quietly to sleep despite having intolerable pain, I do not think any problem would have arisen. It is because he gave her a particular substance intravenously which could have no other consequence than to stop her heart that he was charged and convicted' (p. 117).[2]

Seedhouse and Lovett argue that although the notion of double effect 'can be of great psychological help to a carer who has to make this sort of choice, it is of dubious philosophical validity' (p. 50).[3]

As you may have already gathered, the BMA does not explicitly share this scepticism of the doctrine. The BMA writes: 'The BMA and the law embrace the principle of double-effect, which provides justification for provision of medical treatment that has bad effects when the intention is to provide an overall good effect' (p. 391).[1]

Sanctity of life

Some people argue that human life is of absolute value. Life, they claim, is something which must be preserved at all costs, whatever its quality. However, most people do not give life this extreme sanctity (although they may ascribe *some* intrinsic value to life) and the law accepts that there are some situations in which life is not worth living.

Very few people believe that all forms of life are sacred. In the case of human life, biological life can be distinguished from biographical life. **Biological life** is the **presence of vital signs** whereas **biographical life** is life that **has a meaning.** Tony Bland after the Hillsborough disaster had biological life without biographical life: he could not communicate, had no taste, no sense of smell, no feelings of pleasure or distress. Few people would consider such a life to be worth living, and even people who argue that vital signs have intrinsic value need to balance this with other considerations, such as the avoidance of suffering.

As I write this, Mr Justice Hedley has just announced his verdict on the case of Charlotte Wyatt, an 11-month-old, severely disabled baby who was born three months premature. The doctors, on the basis of her constant suffering, poor quality of life, and terrible prognosis, decided to allow Charlotte to die if she required resuscitation, as she had done three times previously. Charlotte's parents, both devout Christians, disagreed with the doctors' decision and took the case to court. Justice Hedley backed the doctors and ruled that Charlotte should be allowed to die if her condition deteriorates.

In his judgment, Justice Hedley said: "I do not believe that any further aggressive treatment, even if necessary to prolong life, is in her best interests. [...] I believe and find that further invasive and aggressive treatment would be intolerable to Charlotte".[4] So, even if one ascribes some intrinsic value to life, a life racked with pain and suffering may have greater **disvalue** than the intrinsic value of life itself. Note, however, that people's interpretation of 'value' and 'disvalue' can differ! These are not objective terms.

What counts as suffering?

In most debates on euthanasia, the arguments involve discussion of severe physical pain or disability and their impact on a person's self-worth. However, the devastating effects of mental suffering also deserve attention. In the 1990s, Dr Chabot, a Dutch psychiatrist, assisted the suicide of a 50-year-old woman whose two sons had died and who had been beaten by her alcoholic husband. She told Dr Chabot that she no longer wished to live. The Dutch Supreme Court found that, although free from terminal illness, she was suffering greatly. Thus, they considered the assisted suicide lawful. This case demonstrated that perhaps it is **the degree of suffering that matters, rather than its origin.** Mental pain can be as unbearable as physical pain.

The 'killing versus letting die' distinction

Is there a moral difference between killing someone and letting someone die? Legally, such a distinction is pivotal to the legal acceptability of passive euthanasia and the unacceptability of active euthanasia or physician assisted suicide. However, the concepts of killing and letting die are vague. It is generally accepted that **killing** is a **causal action** which **brings about death,** whereas **letting die** is the **intentional avoidance of action,** so that disease causes death. The *acts/omissions distinction* states that there may be a moral difference between actively doing something and omitting to do something, even if both result in the same consequences. Killing can be thought of as an act, whereas letting die is an omission. Therefore, under the acts/omissions distinction, killing is morally worse than letting die (all other things being equal).

However, it is difficult to draw a line between acts and omissions. For example, removing nutrition so that the patient dies can be both killing (an act) and letting die (an omission). Perhaps deliberately not doing something is an act in itself (i.e. the act of doing nothing)! The moral distinctions between active and passive euthanasia, however, rest largely on there being a fundamental difference between acts and omissions. For many people, active euthanasia, which involves an act of killing, is morally worse than passive euthanasia, which involves an omission resulting in death.

Intuitively, there does seem to be a difference between acts and omissions. After all, it would be odd to hold me responsible for the hundreds of sudanese famine victims I failed to save by not giving to charity.

Sometimes, however, the distinction is blurred, as some acts of letting die count as killing. A thought experiment by Beauchamp and Childress illustrates how the morality of killing or letting die is not based on the type of action itself, and how the boundaries between the two categories are not always clear cut.

> **The two patients on a ventilator**
> *Imagine two patients in a hospital room. Both have exactly the same illness and are dependent on respirators to stay alive. The first patient has refused the respirator, whereas the second patient wants to stay connected. A doctor comes in and intentionally flicks the master switch which turns off both respirators. Both patients die in exactly the same way.*[5]
>
> Although both died of the same physical causes and by the same action, their deaths are different from the point of view of morality. The doctor unjustifiably killed one person (the patient who wanted to remain on the respirator), but justifiably let the other die. What justifies the action, therefore, is not whether it was killing or letting die, but whether the patient gave a **valid authorisation** for the action. It is this which makes the action right or wrong.

Gillon supports the view of Beauchamp and Childress when he argues that there is 'no morally relevant difference between acts as a class and omissions as a class, and, in particular, between [...] actions described as killings and [...] omissions described as letting die'.[6]

Ordinary versus extraordinary means

The distinction between ordinary and extraordinary means is sometimes used to justify forgoing life-saving or life-sustaining treatment. The idea behind the distinction is this: it is **morally acceptable to forgo extraordinary treatments but it is *not* acceptable to forgo ordinary treatments.** Roman Catholic theologians used the distinction to decide whether a refusal of treatment was suicide: if you refused an extraordinary treatment, then you did not commit suicide, but if you refused ordinary treatment, you did!

There are several problems with the distinction. Beauchamp and Childress call the distinction 'unacceptably vague and morally misleading' (p. 123).[5] **How do we decide which treatments are ordinary and which are extraordinary?** Is an extraordinary treatment, for example, one that is rarely performed, one that is very expensive, one that is highly invasive, one that is complex, one that is risky, or something else entirely? Furthermore, there is no logical link between the (medical) ordinariness of a medical treatment and the morality of its use. This depends on the circumstances, including the patient's wishes. It may be morally desirable to stop giving a patient antibiotics, for example, if this will only prolong an unbearable life (think of a variant of the Baby Wyatt case mentioned earlier). The decision to treat a patient should depend on a number of factors, not merely the ordinariness or extraordinariness of a treatment. Beauchamp and Childress conclude that the distinction between ordinary versus extraordinary means 'should be replaced by the distinction between **optional and obligatory** treatment, as determined by the balance of benefits and burdens to the patient' (p. 125).[5]

'Do Not Resuscitate' (DNR) orders

What is a DNR order?

A DNR order (sometimes called a Do Not Attempt to Resuscitate (DNAR) order) is a **decision that cardiopulmonary resuscitation (CPR) will not be attempted if the patient requires resuscitation.**

Resuscitation should be considered a treatment like any other. Like all treatments, the doctor is not obliged to provide the treatment if it is deemed futile or not in the patient's best interests, *even if the patient requests it.* As there is no proxy consent for adults in English law, **family members can neither demand nor refuse resuscitation on behalf of the patient.**

When should doctors consider a DNR decision?

1. If resuscitation is likely to be **futile**.

2. If a competent patient has given a **valid refusal** of resuscitation (note that resuscitating a patient who has given a valid refusal constitutes **battery**).

3. If resuscitation will lead to a quality of life so low that the procedure would **not be in the patient's best interests.**

What do we mean by 'futile'?

In some cases, it is obvious that a treatment is futile. If a patient is dead, no amount of antibiotics will help his recovery! Yet the concept of futility is not always clear. Does futility refer only to the statistical chances of a procedure's success, or does it have an evaluative component to it? (i.e. people have to decide whether the benefits of a procedure outweigh the burdens). As Hope, Savulescu and Hendrick suggest, it appears to be a combination of both (p. 167).[7] In other words, people may disagree over what constitutes 'futility'. You might consider a 1% chance of survival futile, but I might not. Even if we both accept that the chance of a successful outcome is 1%, we may weigh up the burdens and benefits of the treatment differently. This would be an argument for allowing patients to decide whether or not a treatment was futile. The main problem with this is cost. Respecting the wishes of a patient who wants to live at all costs may be extremely expensive and divert limited resources away from other areas.

> **In practice:** DNR orders should be documented in the patient's medical records by the most senior member of the available medical team. The doctor in charge should also note the reasons for the decision and whether any relatives were involved in the decision. DNR decisions should be **reviewed regularly**.

Death certification and the role of the coroner's court

Doctors attending patients during their final illness must sign a *Medical Certificate of the Cause of Death* (MCCD), record the cause of death, and send the certificate to the local Registrar of Births, Deaths and Marriages. If the doctor was not present during the patient's final illness, if the patient died under anaesthetic or while undergoing an operation, or if the death requires further investigation, the doctor must inform the coroner. The role of the coroner, who is either a lawyer or a doctor, is to *ascertain the medical cause of death*. A coroner may decide to arrange an autopsy or hold an inquest before certifying a death. An inquest is *not* a trial, but an inquiry into the facts surrounding a death.

A doctor may certify the cause of death if:

1. He has seen the patient during the 14 days before death, or

2. He has seen and examined the body after death.

If a doctor does not fulfil these criteria, he must report the death to the coroner.

If the body is to be cremated, the certification process is more elaborate (for the obvious reason that the body cannot be examined later!). A representative of the family needs to fill in a cremation form, the doctor who signed the death certificate should complete another form, and a *second doctor* is required to fill an additional certificate after a) seeing the body and b) talking to the first doctor. (p. 10)[8]

At the time of writing, the doctors who counter-signed death certificates signed by Harold Shipman are under investigation. Seven doctors who worked with Dr Shipman are to face charges of serious professional misconduct by the GMC. The inquiry also concluded that the death certification system should be 'radically reformed'. The appeal court judge chairing the inquiry, Dame Janet Smith, reported that 'all the Hyde doctors now accept that, if they had questioned a relative or person with knowledge of the death, they would in many cases have discovered facts which would have caused them to refuse to sign Form C [the confirmatory medical certificate]'.[9]

More generally, the GMC comments:

> Registered medical practitioners have the authority to sign a variety of documents, such as death certificates, on the assumption that they will only sign statements they believe to be true. This means that you must *take reasonable steps to verify any statements* before you sign a document. You must not sign documents which you believe to be false or misleading.10

Note that there is a difference between **certifying** a death and **confirming** a death. Whereas only doctors can certify deaths, any health professional can confirm a death.

> **In practice:** If you or a senior colleague are unsure about the cause of death, you should refer the case to the coroner.

Organ transplantation

The ethical and legal issues surrounding organ transplantation are complex. As the life expectancy of the population rises and the waiting list times for organs increase, the field of transplantation ethics is gaining in importance. In this brief section, we will only point out the main ethical issues and expose the relevant law. Should you wish to know more about the subject, we have suggested several excellent articles and books on the subject at the end of the section.

The list of questions below gives an idea of the sorts of issues raised by organ transplantation:

• In light of the shortage of organs, should we change from an 'opt-in' to an 'opt-out' ('presumed consent') system, as is the case in Austria and Belgium? In other words, should we make people register their objection to donating their organs post-mortem?

• What role should relatives have in the decision to use a person's organs. As it stands, **relatives can veto a decision to remove a person's organs for transplantation,** even if the deceased person wanted to donate an organ. The Department of Health states: 'in practice any objections raised by relatives usually take priority over donor's wishes'.[11]

• What is the best way to allocate the insufficient number of organs available? In the UK, organ allocation is controlled by UK Transplant, which aims to allocate the organs in the most fair, unbiased and efficient way. Although the aim is laudable, it is too nebulous to be of any use. The difficult question is: 'what is a fair and unbiased way?'. Is the age of the patient the most important factor, or is it the years they are expected to gain from the transplant? Should a person who smokes, drinks, and eats fast food three time a day be given a heart transplant? As it stands, organs are allocated on the basis of **geographical proximity** between the donor and the hospital treating the recipient, the **chances of success, age** (those under 18 are given priority), and the difference in age between donor and recipient.[7]

• Should people ever be allowed to pay for organs? What are the arguments for and against a commercial market in organs?

• Who should be allowed to become a living donor? Should parents decide whether a very young child should give an organ to a brother or sister? Is it an individual's right to sell their own organs?

What are the laws governing organ donation and transplantation?
There are two Acts of particular relevance.

The Human Tissue Act (1961)
The Act allows the removal of organs from dead persons for transplantation, medical education or research where:

1. Prior to his death, the person expressed a request (in writing or orally in front of two or more witnesses during his last illness) that he wished to donate his body or part of it for medical purposes, or

2. There is no reason to believe that the dead person, even if he did not express a request, did not want his body to be used in this way or withdrew a decision to donate his body before his death, or

3. A surviving spouse or relative does not object to the removal of the body part.

There is no need to ask every single relative for permission to remove the organ. The Department of Health states that 'in most instances it will be sufficient to discuss the matter with any one relative who had been in close contact with the deceased, determining whether there is reason to believe that any other relative would be likely to object'.[11]

The Human Organ Transplants Act (1989)
The Act makes the commercial use of organs for transplantation a criminal offence. Advertising the buying or selling of organs, whether to the public or to a single individual, is also illegal. The Act also makes illegal the transplanting of organs from living donors to recipients who are not genetically related. If a living donor wishes to donate an organ to a non-genetically related recipient (e.g. a spouse), this must be approved by the Unrelated Live Transplant Regulatory Authority (ULTRA).

Further reading:

- Radcliffe-Richards J, Daar A, Guttmann R, Hoffenberg R, Kennedy I, Lock M, et al. The case for allowing kidney sales. *The Lancet* 1998;351(9120):1950-1952.[12]

- Veatch R. *Transplantation ethics*. Washington, D.C.: Georgetown University Press, 2000.[13]

- Caplan A, Coelho D, editors. *The ethics of organ transplants: the current debate*. Amherst, N.Y.: Prometheus, 1999.[14]

- Wilkinson S. *Bodies for sale: ethics and exploitation in the human body trade*. London: Routledge, 2003.[15]

Summary

- Active euthanasia and physician assisted suicide are **illegal**.

- Passive euthanasia is **not necessarily illegal**.

- The distinctions between acts and omissions, and ordinary and extraordinary means **are conceptually problematic**.

- Resuscitation should be seen as a treatment like any other. Doctors need not resuscitate if a) it is deemed **futile,** b) the patient **validly refuses** to be resuscitated or c) it would **not** be **in the patient's best interests.**

- DNR orders should be **documented in the patient's notes** by the senior doctor and **reviewed regularly**.

- Doctors certifying deaths should report any suspicious or unexplainable deaths to the coroner.

- Organ donation and transplantation are regulated by the **Human Tissue Act** (1961) and the **Human Organ Transplants Act** (1989).

References

1. British Medical Association; Medical Ethics Today. London: BMJ Publishing Group, 2004.

2. Dunnett A. *Euthanasia: The Heart of the Matter.* London: Hodder and Stoughton Ltd., 1999.

3. Seedhouse D, Lovett L. *Practical Medical Ethics.* Chichester: John Wiley and Sons Ltd., 1992.

4. 'The issue is not whether this baby should die but how and when'. *The Times* 2004;6.

5. Beauchamp T, Childress J. *Principles of Biomedical Ethics.* 5th ed. Oxford: Oxford University Press, 2001.

6. Gillon R. Acts and omissions, killing and letting die. *British Medical Journal* 1986;292(6513):126-127.

7. Hope T, Savulescu J, Hendrick J. *Medical ethics and law: the core curriculum.* Edinburgh: Churchill Livingstone, 2003.

8. Death certification and investigation in England, Wales and Northern Ireland – The report of a fundamental review 2003. Presented to Parliament by the Secretary of State for the Home Department by Command of Her Majesty. London, 2003.

9. Death certification and the investigation of deaths by coroners, 2003.

10. General Medical Council: Good Medical Practice 'Signing certificates and other documents'.

11. Code of practice for the diagnosis of brain stem death. London: Department of Health, 1998:HSC 1998/035.

12. Radcliffe-Richards J, Daar A, Guttmann R, Hoffenberg R, Kennedy I, Lock M, et al. The case for allowing kidney sales. *The Lancet* 1998;351(9120):1950-1952.

13. Veatch R. *Transplantation ethics*. Washington, D.C.: Georgetown University Press, 2000.

14. Caplan A, Coelho D, editors. *The ethics of organ transplants: the current debate*. Amherst, N.Y.: Prometheus, 1999.

15. Wilkinson S. *Bodies for sale: ethics and exploitation in the human body trade*. London: Routledge, 2003.

Survival and sanity: vulnerabilities created by the duties of doctors and medical students

Medicine is a rewarding and challenging profession. It is also immensely stressful, particularly at a time when public expectations are high and patients are increasingly willing to challenge what they are told.

The stresses that doctors face on a daily basis can cause physical, mental and emotional problems, which may affect their performance at work. This chapter looks at some of the vulnerabilities faced by doctors and medical students. It covers medical mistakes, poor performance, issues around doctors' health, GMC regulation, and how to deal with commonly encountered problems. It includes advice from the MPS on handling complaints and a section entitled 'Coalface ethics and the junior doctor', which illustrates the reality of ethical problems in everyday practice.

Common dilemmas for medical students

Medical students can face unique difficulties in their day-to-day lives. The patients you meet are often seriously ill and under great stress. Balancing your own need to learn without offending patients or upsetting a busy clinical team can be delicate. Most medical students are used to feeling clumsy, ignorant and constantly in the way. There are also the thorny issues of learning practical skills and interacting with senior doctors. You know that learning how to insert a venflon is vital for the care of your future patients, but you still suffer pangs of guilt for the first patients subjected to your inept attempts at cannulation. Many of us have squirmed uncomfortably when introduced by consultants as a 'junior doctor', whilst wearing a badge reading 'MEDICAL STUDENT' in inch-high letters.

What are the main ethical issues concerning medical students?

The BMA Medical Students Committee has compiled a list of ethical issues relevant to medical students (p. 669)[1]. These include:

- How students should be **introduced** to patients.

- Patient **consent** to student involvement in consultations and treatment.

- **Inexperience** in carrying out procedures.

- **Conflicts** between furthering your medical education and caring for the patient.

- Carrying out **intimate examinations** on anaesthetised patients.

And what to do when:

- You believe that senior colleagues have impaired judgement.

- You believe you have witnessed poor practice.

- You know that fellow students are acting incompetently or dangerously.

We have already addressed some of these issues earlier in the book. For example, the proper introduction of medical students to patients and the requirements for consent are discussed in chapter 2. Issues surrounding intimate examinations on anaesthetised patients are examined in the article 'How to be a good medical student', also in chapter 2. The other concerns are discussed below.

Thankfully, as students we do not have to take full responsibility for making decisions (and, as doctors, our responsibility will increase gradually with experience). This means we can, and usually should, **seek advice** from a clinical tutor or senior colleague when uncertain. However, a student who has genuine concerns about a senior colleague may be in an even more difficult position than a doctor.

As a medical student, you are dependent on senior colleagues and teachers to progress through medical school. The people that teach you now will write your references and may even determine whether you pass the course. You might end up working under them after you qualify. For these reasons, students often feel unable to speak out, even if convinced that a senior colleague has acted incorrectly.

What should I do if I think a senior doctor has acted inappropriately?

If you are concerned about a doctor's actions, there are a few points to consider before taking things further:

1. There are very real **differences in knowledge** between students and experienced clinicians. Students should always question their perception of poor practice before taking action.

2. Do you know all the **facts** about the case? There may be relevant aspects to the case that for some reason have not been shared with the student.

3. There will always be disagreements over the best way to manage patients. Often, there may be **several valid approaches.** The most experienced doctor with overall responsibility for the patient has to decide between them.

Nevertheless, there may be occasions where students do witness dubious conduct by a senior doctor. If you believe that 'following orders' will harm patients, or if what you see is seriously at odds with what you have been taught, then you **have a duty to make these concerns known.**

Who should I tell?

First, you should ask the doctor in question why they made that decision or chose to manage the patient in that way. If done in a non-confrontational way, this should not cause offence. After all, medical students are encouraged to understand and question why things are done. This should also help clarify matters if you have misunderstood or overlooked something.

If no explanation is given, or if you still have concerns, you might want to take things further:

- Again, the first step should be to **express your concern** to the doctor in question in a sensitive and non-confrontational way.

- Sometimes this may not be possible, or you might not be convinced by the answer. In this case, you should **follow local procedures.** This means following the guidelines of your medical school for dealing with such issues. For example, can you speak to a personal tutor or mentor about the situation?

- It may be a good idea to **share your concerns** with a trusted fellow student to see if he agrees with your evaluation.

- If still in doubt, you should consider seeking advice from a senior colleague.

Similar guidelines apply to the dubious conduct of fellow medical students. If you believe that patient care may suffer you must speak out. All medical schools should have internal procedures for dealing with such matters.

Practical Procedures – what should I do if I feel out of my depth?

I have learned since to be a better student, and to be ready to say to my fellow students "I do not know." [2] William Osler

From time to time, we are asked to do things that we don't feel comfortable doing. As a medical student, you still have the luxury to decline the offer. If you don't feel comfortable doing a procedure on a patient, don't do it! It may be embarrassing to admit in front of the whole ward-round that you don't know how to remove a venflon, but it's a lot less unpleasant than doing something against your will, or explaining to a patient why you made a mistake. Don't be embarrassed to **ask for help.** It is better to ask now, as an ignorant student, than as an ignorant PRHO!

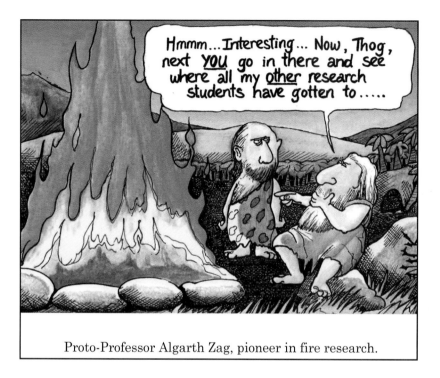

Proto-Professor Algarth Zag, pioneer in fire research.

Responsibilities and vulnerabilities after qualification

What is the role of the General Medical Council?

The GMC was established by the Medical Act of 1858. It is a self-regulatory body composed of doctors and lay persons. The functions of the GMC include:

- **Maintaining and revalidating the register of all medical practitioners.**
  The GMC holds a register which lists all the doctors qualified to practise medicine in the UK. If you are removed from the register, you may no longer practise medicine legally. Removal (i.e. getting 'struck off') is the ultimate sanction that the GMC can impose. Traditionally, once qualified, doctors remained on the register for life. Their right to practise was only re-examined if questions arose about their performance. This is no longer the case today. From 1 April 2005, all doctors will have to demonstrate regularly to the GMC that their knowledge and skills are up to date and that they are still fit to practise ('revalidation').[3]

- **Setting standards** for behaviour and **issuing guidance** to support doctors and protect patients, e.g. the GMC guidelines *'duties of a doctor'*.

- **Investigating complaints about the conduct, performance or health of doctors.** Doctors, patients, relatives or employers can complain to the GMC about a doctor's conduct or performance. The Police also notify the GMC if a doctor is convicted of a criminal offence.

The GMC is responsible for **issuing sanctions** to doctors found guilty of misconduct or poor performance. Depending on the gravity of the offence, the GMC can:

1. Caution a doctor.

2. Impose conditions on a doctor's registration.

3. Suspend registration.

4. Remove a doctor from the medical register.

What is the difference between misconduct, poor performance and negligence?

Misconduct is the **deliberate failure** to follow professional standards. This is rare, but is usually very serious when it does occur.

Poor performance is when doctors unintentionally produce substandard care. It may result from working under stressful or disorganised conditions.

Poor performance will affect many doctors at some point in their careers. Over 5% of senior hospital doctors will have performance problems in any 5-year period. Between 30 and 40 PRHOs and SHOs are referred annually to postgraduate deans for serious behaviour, performance or mental health problems.[4]

Negligence is different again to poor performance and misconduct. The concept of negligence was introduced in chapter 2. A doctor can be found guilty of negligence if:

1. The doctor had a **duty of care** to the patient and **failed in that duty**, and

2. This **caused harm** to the patient (physical or psychological).

Patients who have suffered from medical error can sue doctors for negligence through the civil courts. For a full reminder of the law on negligence, see chapter 2.

What shall I do when a colleague has performance problems?

Although junior doctors are often among the first to recognise performance problems in colleagues, they may be reluctant to speak out, perhaps through loyalty or for fear of damaging their careers. However, **doctors have a duty to intervene** to protect both the health of the doctor concerned and the safety of patients.

If you believe that a colleague is putting patients at risk, the GMC recommends **explaining your concerns** to the appropriate person in the employing authority (e.g. the Medical Director). You should follow **local guidelines** as discussed earlier in relation to students. Again, if you are not happy with the response, you may want to take further action. In serious cases, this may include **informing the GMC.** You can always contact the GMC or your defence body for advice.

Whistleblowing

The term 'whistleblowing' refers to people who expose misconduct or poor practice in the workplace. The Public Interest Disclosure Act (1998) was set up to encourage more people to report malpractice at work. It protects those (the 'whistleblowers') who draw attention to malpractice, as long as the disclosure is done in 'good faith'. In certain circumstances, 'whistleblowers' may justifiably inform the police or the media if they:

• Reasonably believe they would be **victimised** if they raised the concern internally, or with a prescribed regulator.

• Believe a **cover-up** is likely, or if there is no prescribed regulator.

• Have raised the matter internally or with a prescribed regulator and **no satisfactory action was taken.**

If whistleblowers are victimised as a result of their disclosure they can seek compensation through an employment tribunal. If sacked, they can apply for an interim order to keep their job. The 'whistleblowing' legislation may offer some protection if you suffer adverse consequences as a result of speaking out.

As previously mentioned, always follow **local procedures** first. It is also advisable to **consult your defence union** before taking any action.

Mistakes in medical practice

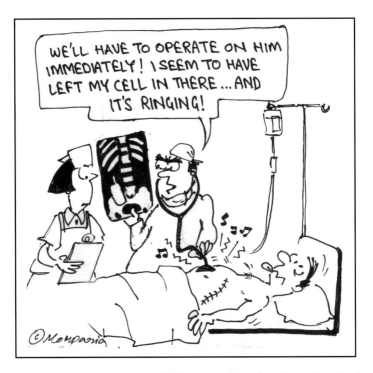

A **mistake** is an *unintentional* error of judgement. A harsh reality of medical practice is that all doctors **will make mistakes at some point**. 'The wisest of the wise may err', as the ancient Greek playwright, Aeschylus, wrote. In medicine, the smallest mistake can have tragic consequences. But the *consequences* of that error will depend not only on the mistake itself, but also on our *response* to the mistake and the *environment* in which it is carried out. It is the job of the individual doctor and of the system in which he works to reduce the impact of error by:

1. Attempting to **minimize** mistakes and their **consequences**.

2. Knowing how to **respond** to mistakes.

3. **Learning** from them.

True story: Reducing the impact of unanticipated errors in clinical practice[5]

An elderly woman was admitted to hospital for surgery on her right hand, which was marked with a water-soluble marker. In the hours before the operation, the woman sat with her arms folded. During the wait, the mark on her right hand rubbed off onto her left.

While in the anaesthetic room, doctors checked the consent form for the procedure. Fortunately, despite the presence of the marker pen on the left side, they noticed that consent for surgery had been given for the opposite hand. The operation was thus performed on the correct hand.

Surprising fact: 1/5 of American hand surgeons say they have operated on the wrong hand at some point in their career. (p. 9)[6]

Conclusion: The case above illustrates the need to be vigilant to potential error, and to always check and recheck the details before carrying out a risky procedure.

While some errors are unavoidable, doctors can take steps to reduce the likelihood of mistakes or poor performance (p. 736):[1]

- Always work within the limits of your professional competence.

- Keep your knowledge and skills up to date.

- Maintain good communication within the medical team and with the patient.

- Take part in clinical audit and respond to the outcomes of reviews, assessments and appraisals.

- Be aware of changing social expectations.

- Be aware of the performance of colleagues.

True story: A fatal medical mistake[7]

A 16-year-old patient was undergoing chemotherapy treatment for leukaemia. He attended hospital monthly for intravenous injections of Vincristine, with additional injections of intrathecal methotrexate every other month.

In February 1990, he attended for both injections. The hospital pharmacy sent up the injections to the ward in a red box, and these were placed on a trolley set up for the lumbar puncture. The name of each drug and relevant method of administration was clearly marked on the box and on each syringe.

The House Officer asked to perform the procedure was reluctant to do so due to his inexperience. An SHO was sent to supervise him. The House Officer injected the Vincristine (rather than the intended methotrexate) into the patient's CSF under the supervision of the SHO.

Why did this happen? This error arose because the HO thought that the SHO was supervising the whole procedure, whereas the SHO assumed he was supervising only the lumbar puncture. The SHO handed the HO the wrong syringe. **Poor communication** undoubtedly played a major role in this error.

The consequences: Sadly, this mistake resulted in the death of the patient. Both doctors were convicted of manslaughter. They were given suspended prison sentences, but the convictions were overturned on appeal. The lessons from this tragedy have still not been learnt. Several similar deaths from erroneous administration of Vincristine into the CSF have recently occurred in the UK.

What could be done to prevent this happening again: Any number of simple measures would help, for example:

- Specialist training in cytotoxic drug therapy for doctors needing to administer it.

- Never administering more than one drug at a time.

- Careful checking and rechecking of drugs by more than one colleague.

- Changing the design of the syringe used for Vincristine, so that it cannot be used for intrathecal administration.

It's acceptable to say sorry

Some medical students and doctors feel anxious about apologising to patients for their mistakes. They may feel that saying sorry is an admission of guilt, leaving them legally liable. This is not true. An apology is **not** an admission of culpability, and saying sorry can be of great comfort to the patient. Most patients will accept that mistakes happen occasionally. They may be more upset by the deception involved in disguising an error, than by the error itself.

Patients who have been involved in mistakes are entitled to receive a full and honest account of what went wrong and the likely consequences for their health. While this may be difficult, it is absolutely essential. Patients should know about mistakes to obtain any future care needed as a result. They may also wish to seek compensation for their injuries. Having said this, a courteous apology and full explanation of why things went wrong may actually reduce the likelihood of the patient making a formal complaint or taking legal action against you.

Once any acute or emergency medical care issues are dealt with, it is helpful to discuss the events with more senior colleagues. Ideally, you should speak to the consultant with overall responsibility for the patient. The consultant may wish to speak to the patient himself, or be present when you do. In any case, he must be aware of the incident. Depending on the mistake, a more experienced doctor may be in a better position to put the mistake in context, particularly with regard to the possible health consequences.

Preventing the recurrence of mistakes

In recent years there has been a great desire to change the 'blame culture' pervading the medical profession. In an ideal world there would be an open, non-judgmental environment in which people could discuss their mistakes and near-misses. Colleagues could learn from each other's experiences and the system could be improved to prevent their recurrence. However, achieving this would require a shift in thinking on the part of patients and the wider public. They would need to accept that some uncertainties and errors are inevitable (p. 759).[1] An anonymous national reporting system, the National Patient Safety Agency, was set up in 2001 as a means of reporting mistakes (see Appendix C for contact details).

What causes doctors to make mistakes?

Whilst individual error may play a role, most errors are caused by a combination of factors, such as staff shortage, poor communication, or stressful working conditions. A 1998 BMA report on work-related stress amongst junior doctors listed the main problems as:

• **Stress:** excessive workload and long hours.

• **Fatigue.**

• **Covering** for sick colleagues with insufficient locum support.

• **A professional culture** that prevents doctors from using formal support services.

• Feeling that they have to **make decisions alone:** an unspoken pressure not to call on senior staff especially during antisocial hours.

• Feeling **unable to admit to uncertainty** for fear of appearing incompetent or damaging job prospects (p. 745).[1]

Long working hours and lack of support undoubtedly contribute to performance problems. There may be some improvement in these areas in the next few years, with the introduction of the European Working Time Directive and initiatives such as the 'Hospital at Night' project.[8] Yet there will always be some degree of stress inherent in the job. Doctors also need to take responsibility for aspects of their own performance or character that could contribute to error, such as illness or an unwillingness to seek help.

Sickness amongst doctors, their colleagues, family and friends

The pressures of long hours, disturbed sleep, dealing with patient suffering, and alienation from family and friends can take a heavy toll on a doctor's health. It can lead to burnout, mental health problems and a reliance on alcohol and drugs. Depression, anxiety and substance misuse are well documented among doctors, and many may not be getting the support they need.

Doctors are twice as likely to be depressed as the general population. Male doctors are twice as likely, and female doctors three to four times as likely to commit suicide than non-medics.[9] More than two-thirds of cases considered by the GMC's Health Committee in 2002 involved the misuse of drugs and alcohol, and roughly one in fifteen doctors in the UK suffers from some form of dependence.[10]

Traditionally, doctors have overlooked or underplayed their own health problems. One reason may be that doctors feel guilty about taking sick leave as it puts pressure on their colleagues. They may worry about confidentiality issues when seeking help, especially if suffering from mental health problems. However, mental health services are used to having doctors as patients. Depression, anxiety and alcoholism are treatable conditions. It is now usually possible to ask for an **out of area referral** for mental health problems. Often, doctors with mental health problems can continue to practise whilst undergoing treatment if supervised and following an agreed treatment plan.

Doctors are also entitled to be treated fairly with respect to disability or chronic illness. Disabled doctors are exposed to additional vulnerabilities and may require support. An example of such a service is the BMA's chronic illness matching scheme. This gives doctors suffering from chronic illness a chance to meet other doctors in the same situation.[9] An extension of the Disability Discrimination Act (DDA) 1995 came into force on 1 October 2004 and may further protect doctors against unfair discrimination.

What should you do if sick?

As a doctor, you are responsible for ensuring that your own health does not have a detrimental effect on patient care. The best policy is to:

- Register with your **own GP.**

- **Avoid informal 'corridor' consultations.** These can be uncomfortable for both you and your colleague. Besides, your colleague may not be the best placed person to give you optimum care.

- **Act promptly** on early warning signs if something is wrong.

There are a number of support services available, including over-the-phone advice and support.

Some support services:

- Doctors Support Line: 'staffed by volunteer doctors to provide peer support for doctors and medical students in the UK'. Tel 0870 7650001 www.doctorssupport.org

- National Counselling Service for Sick Doctors: 24 hour helpline 0870 2410535, www.ncssd.org.uk

- The BMA Counselling Service: tel 0845 9200169 (BMA members only)

What should you do when you're sick?

If you suspect you've been exposed to a serious communicable disease (e.g. HIV, Hep B, Tuberculosis) you must **seek expert advice** from a consultant in Occupational Health, Public Health or Infectious Diseases. You should **never** rely on your own assessment of risk to others.[11] In many cases, doctors will be allowed to continue to work, but advice is needed on any necessary limitations to normal practice.

Certainly, it is not advisable to self-medicate or rely on the informal advice of a colleague. Remember William Osler's dictum: 'a doctor who treats himself has a fool for a patient'. Self-medication can be hazardous and sick doctors may lose insight into the dangers of working when ill. Failure to seek appropriate help early enough may put your long-term health and career prospects at risk. Doctors have the same right to care and support as any other patients.

Avoid treating your family and friends

From your first few weeks of medical school, family and friends have probably been asking for your expert opinion on all sorts of problems. The usual line of defence – "but I haven't done that bit yet!" – will be useless once you qualify. Despite many years of study, it is generally best not to treat your family or friends. There are good reasons for this advice. It may be hard to keep the right **emotional distance** when treating family members and you may also **fail to notice signs** that a dispassionate observer would spot.

After dealing with seriously ill patients all day, it can be tempting to reassure your hypochondriacal mother that there is nothing really wrong with her. However, you would feel terrible if it did turn out to be serious. In rare cases, doctors treating family members could have a conflict of interest. A doctor who stands to inherit from a relative's death could be accused of neglect, for example. **The GMC therefore recommends not treating yourself or family members except in an emergency.**[12] Obviously it's fine to give advice to family members, but it's also wise to encourage them to consult their own doctors if they are worried about something.

Dealing with complaints

All users of the health service are encouraged to make complaints if dissatisfied with the care they have received. Therefore, it is likely that you will receive a number of complaints during your career. Knowing how to deal with complaints is critical.

How shall I deal with a complaint? Guidance from the MPS[13]

The days when doctors were so revered that no one dared complain are long gone. The **best doctors in all specialities** now run the risk of facing a complaint or claim during their career. As a general rule, the experience of the MPS suggests that a GP in full time practice will face one clinical negligence claim in his career. In Ireland, obstetricians/gynaecologists get sued, on average, twice every three years. This means that they will face 20-25 claims throughout their medical career.

Doctors who face a complaint often find that this affects their confidence and their job satisfaction. Many consider the complaint as a personal attack and feel hurt, angry or betrayed.

If you do receive a complaint or a claim, there are certain steps that you should take to help yourself:

- **Don't ignore it.** It won't go away and you could make the situation significantly worse if you don't take action.

- If a patient complains about you, **try not to react defensively.** Don't dismiss it or make counter threats as this will only make things worse.

- If the complaint involves a number of different healthcare professionals, don't be tempted to **shift the blame** onto others.

- **Contact your protection organisation** as soon as you think there may be a problem. The MPS and other protection organisations can give you practical help in dealing with the complaint as well as emotional support if needed.

- **Try to assess the circumstances realistically.** It is easy to blow things out of proportion and let it dominate your whole life.

- **Talk the situation through** with a trusted friend or colleague who can be sympathetic but also give you a realistic assessment of the situation.

- **Inform the relevant person** at the practice or trust and comply with the complaints procedure. The Trust will have policies for dealing with complaints and claims.

- Try to **keep things in perspective.** Remind yourself of the majority of times when you have got things right and helped patients who were grateful for your care.

- **Make notes of the incident** as soon as you believe that there may be a problem. Include any extra details that you won't have put in the patient's notes such as witnesses, anything that may have distracted you at the time of the mistake and, if possible, why you made the decisions that you did.

- **Gather together any relevant documentation.** If things are not immediately resolved it is likely that the trust or your protection organisation will request to see this.

- If necessary, **be prepared to give the patient a face to face explanation,** an apology and an undertaking that you will take steps to avoid a repetition of the problem. Many patients who pursue doctors through the civil courts say they were driven to it because the apology they wanted was never offered. In many cases, the patient will be satisfied with an apology and a full explanation of what went wrong.

- If, after the complaint has been investigated, it is found to have no foundation you should **still see the patient and explain the process and outcome.** It is worth trying to find out why the patient made the complaint.

- When it is over, **try to learn from the mistake.** Think about how you would have done things differently, as well as anything you could do to prevent a similar incident in the future. If you have been wrongly accused of making an error, think about why this happened – was it a communication problem?

Remember that some patients have unrealistic expectations of doctors and it is inevitable that you will occasionally disappoint some of your patients.

Coalface ethics and the junior doctor (with Dr Sonya V Babu-Narayan)[14]

As a junior doctor, many of you will face difficult situations involving ethical issues. This section discusses two common scenarios, chosen from many, which a doctor may encounter as a house officer. By pointing out some of the relevant issues, we hope that you will be better prepared to handle such situations when you face them for the first time.

Although many of the ethical and legal issues have been raised in previous parts of the book, it is useful to see how these would apply in practical situations. The cases can also be used as aids to revision. It is a good idea to refer back to the relevant sections of the book if you feel unsure about an ethical or legal point.

Finally, it is worth repeating that junior doctors who encounter ethical problems, such as those outlined below, should seek the advice of a senior doctor if in any doubt about the best course of action.

Case 1
Self discharge

> You are bleeped to the ward because a patient admitted on yesterday's on call shift wishes to self-discharge from the hospital.

Relevant clinical and ethical issues

Although an unplanned discharge may jeopardise the team care plan, a competent adult may legally refuse medical care whatever the risks to himself. The first step, as the doctor on call, is to establish the competency of the patient. Even though the patient may belong to a different team, you are responsible for the patient's care. If the patient is both competent and adequately informed, his wish to refuse treatment should be respected.

Thus, the immediate tasks are:

1. Finding out if the patient is **competent.**

2. Ensuring that the patient is **adequately informed** about his decision to self discharge.

The patient should be informed of any good reasons for staying in the hospital. He may well change his mind; perhaps he was unaware of the severity of his condition, or of the benefits of ongoing admission. Alternatively, he may still decide to leave and, if so, his decision should be respected.

Clinical assessment of competence

There is no perfect, universally accepted way of determining competence but the following questions should be answered:

- Does the patient understand and believe the information given?

- Can the patient weigh such information in a balance and make a choice?

Competence should be established with reference to a particular decision. A patient may be competent to make some decisions but not others. A patient found incompetent yesterday may be competent today. This variability should be kept in mind when assessing the patient. It is also crucial to **document** the assessment of competence and whether the patient has fulfilled the criteria.

Many people believe in a sliding-scale system for establishing competence: the greater the risk, the stricter the criteria for competence. It seems reasonable to be much more stringent in evaluating competence if the patient risks death, for example, than if he risks something pretty harmless. In any case, you should respect the patient's values (even if they may differ from your own) whilst keeping in mind that medical conditions and drug therapies may cause a degree of confusion.

After discussion with the patient and, if possible, the team with overall clinical responsibility, you may be able to reach a compromise, such as allowing the discharge now but with early follow-up.

It deemed appropriate, it may be a good idea to offer the patient a second opinion.

All conversations should be **documented** in detail. This won't be easy to do once the patient has left and you need to rush off to the next urgent problem. Remember: **if you don't document it, it didn't happen!**

Informed choice

As we mentioned earlier, the patient must be given all the necessary information to make an informed decision.

Patience and good communication are essential. If possible, and if the patient agrees, you may want to share the information in the presence of the patient's friend or relative. Once the relevant issues have been explained, the patient may want to reconsider the decision.

Local policy

Most hospitals have a specific form that the patient must complete and sign to indicate that they are leaving hospital against medical advice. The ward nurses will probably be able to help you with this.

Relevant law

The right to refuse treatment, physical or otherwise, is protected by laws against **battery.**

If, however, doctors are satisfied that the patient lacks competence, they may provide treatment in the patient's best interests. In certain cases, this may entail detaining the patient.

The **Mental Health Act** only applies when detaining someone for assessment or treatment of their mental health, not for medical treatment. At the time of going to press, relatives and friends have no legal rights to consent or refuse treatment for adult patients. Still, it is good practice to involve the family in decisions involving incompetent patients.

Case 2
Consenting patients

One night on the ward, you are asked to consent a patient who is scheduled for a procedure early the next morning. The consent form has not yet been signed and ward staff are concerned that this will result in a delay to the list in the morning.

How can you help?

Relevant clinical and ethical issues

Requests to perform tasks for which you feel unsupported

Sometimes, doctors feel obliged to carry out tasks beyond their experience or capabilities. If asked to obtain consent for a procedure you are unfamiliar with, you should not feel pressured to accept. Without an adequate knowledge of the procedure, you may fail to provide the information necessary to allow the patient to make an informed choice.

Amongst other things, you would need to discuss the purpose of the investigation/treatment, the details and uncertainties of the diagnosis, the treatment and non-treatment options, the likely benefits, success, risks, and side effects of the procedure, any possibility of additional problems becoming apparent at the time of the procedure, and the actions that could follow if the problems actually occurred. This requires a fairly detailed knowledge of the procedure!

Most of the time, more experienced colleagues will be available to help us in our tasks and decisions. As long as we are courteous, it is unlikely that our colleagues will decline to help.

Clinical assessment of competence and informed choice

See our discussion in case study 1. Competence is a pre-requisite for valid, informed consent.

Relevant good medical practice guidelines

Check your local and departmental guidelines for the level of risk that should be quoted to patients.

To obtain consent, the GMC guidelines state that the doctor should:

• Be suitably trained and qualified.

• Have **sufficient knowledge** of the proposed investigation or treatment, and understand the risks involved.

• Act in accordance with the guidance in the GMC's *Good Medical Practice* booklet.

The BMA working party recommends that the doctor obtaining consent should be the one recommending the procedure to the patient. In a hospital setting, this would usually be the senior clinician. Reaffirming consent can be done by a delegated junior, as long as he is *suitably trained, qualified and familiar with the procedure*. The doctor who is providing treatment or undertaking the investigation is responsible for ensuring that consent has been obtained.

Relevant law

Patients over 16 are presumed competent to consent unless proved otherwise. See chapter 8 for details of the law on children.

No person, including a relative, can give consent on behalf of an incompetent adult. However, doctors can treat an incompetent adult if they believe treatment is in the patient's best interests. People close to the individual may provide valuable information on some of the relevant non-medical factors, such as the patient's needs and preferences.

If a previously competent adult has indicated that he would refuse all or certain treatments in certain circumstances (i.e. made an 'advance directive'), and those circumstances arise, you are legally required to respect the refusal. The doctor must make sure the directive was made by the person in question, that the patient was competent and informed at the time of making the request, and that the directive applies to the current circumstances. If in doubt, seek legal advice as soon as possible.

Tips

- Maintain good communication with patients and colleagues.

- Try to keep up to date with medical knowledge and skills, as well as guidelines from professional bodies.

- Document your actions in the notes legibly, including the time and whether you sought senior advice or outside help. The importance of good notes will become apparent in 'delicate' legal, ethical or medical situations. A court may assume that 'if you didn't document it, it didn't happen'.

- The GMC and medical defence organisations have helpful websites (see Appendix D).

- If in doubt about something, in particular if it has legal repercussions, run it by someone from your defence organisation or the legal representative in your Trust. There is someone available at all times.

The cases above clearly demonstrate the **practical benefits** of knowing the basics of medical ethics and law. An awareness of the ethical issues that arise in everyday practice will be of great help when dealing with your own problematic situations.

Summary

- A number of stresses and vulnerabilities can impact on the health and performance of doctors.

- Doctors should take proper care of their own health. They should **register with a GP** and avoid self-medication or informal consultations with colleagues.

- Doctors have a **duty to seek help** about underperforming colleagues if they believe patient care might suffer. Local procedures should be followed in the first instance.

- The GMC is responsible for investigating doctors with performance problems.

- Mistakes are unavoidable in medical practice. Doctors should be **vigilant** to avoid unanticipated errors and be aware of the need for **clear communication.**

- Patients who have been affected by mistakes should receive a full explanation and apology. Steps should be put in place to try to **prevent** the **recurrence** of mistakes.

- Doctors should **avoid treating family members or friends** except in an emergency.

- Most importantly, medical students and doctors should not hesitate to **seek help and advice** if in difficulty.

References

1. British Medical Association; Medical Ethics Today. London: BMJ Publishing Group, 2004.

2. Osler W. *Aphorisms from his bedside teachings and writings*. New York: Henry Schuman, Inc, 1950.

3. GMC. Revalidation fact sheet, 2004.

4. Department of Health. Supporting doctors, protecting patients: a consultation paper on preventing, recognising and dealing with the poor clinical performance of doctors in the NHS in England. London, 1999.

5. Butler M, Belcher H. Minerva. *British Medical Journal* 2002;325:1182.

6. Horton R. *Second opinion; doctors, diseases and decisions in modern medicine*. London: Granta Books, 2003.

7. R v Prentice and Sullman 4 Med LR 304, 1993.

8. NHS Modernisation Agency. Findings and recommendations from the Hospital at Night Project., 2004.

9. Graske J. Improving the health of doctors. *British Medical Journal* 2003;337:s188.

10. General Medical Council. Fitness to practise statistics for 2002. London, 2003.

11. General Medical Council. Serious Communicable Diseases.

12. General Medical Council. Doctors should not treat themselves or their families. July 1998. URL: http://www.gmc-uk.org/standards/selftreat.htm

13. This section was modified from material kindly provided by the Medical Protection Society.

14. Thanks to Dr Sonya Babu-Narayan for providing the cases and writing most of the material.

Setting priorities: resource allocation and rationing in healthcare

Why ration?

In an ideal world, everyone in need would get the best medical treatment (assuming disease would exist in such a world!). Alas, in the real world, **resources are finite.** The UK's population is ageing, and costly chronic conditions now make up much of the disease burden. With the availability of new treatments and ever more expensive drugs, resource allocation issues grow more pressing each year. Some kind of 'rationing' is therefore inevitable.

The word 'rationing' is an emotive term. Many people see it as a deliberate attempt to deny some people access to treatment on the grounds of cost alone. But the original meaning of the word 'rationing' (derived from the Latin term *ratio*, meaning rationality), was actually about *rationalising* things and bringing order to chaos.[1] In the context of health care, this means finding a sensible way to **balance scarce resources** with the ever-growing **demands** made upon them. However, there will always be a degree of controversy surrounding any priority setting in the NHS.

Implicit and explicit rationing

To some extent, **implicit** rationing occurs within any healthcare system. For example, patients who live in affluent areas tend to have access to better health facilities than those in poorer areas, despite having less need (this is known as the *inverse care law*). Waiting lists are an indirect way of rationing access to surgical procedures, as some patients will either die, become too sick for the operation, or seek private treatment before reaching the top of the list.

At times, doctors have to explicitly choose who to treat and who not to treat. Traditionally, many rationing decisions have been made locally. Some authors argue that local decision-making is a sensible approach, as it allows consideration of locally important priorities and values.[2] But 'postcode prescribing', as it is sometimes called, has generated much public anger. An inequality of access to treatments (including IVF and beta-interferon), based on geographical location alone, was unpopular with the public, who are seldom told about the criteria used to make decisions at a local level. To reflect this public concern, there is now a greater need for rationing decisions to be both **explicit and justifiable**.[3]

Ethical issues in resource allocation

In many areas of medicine, a doctor's primary concern is for the **patient facing him**. However, when dealing with resource allocation issues, a shift in thinking is needed. Decisions about the treatment of *a particular patient* will have implications for *other patients* within a GP practice, the hospital trust, or indeed nationally.

What do we mean by 'fairness' in resource allocation?

Everyone agrees that scare resources should be distributed **fairly**. But what does fairness mean in this context?

Perhaps the fairest way of allocating goods is to distribute them equally among people (**equality of distribution**). In many areas of life, if all people have an *equal potential to benefit,* we ought to *distribute evenly* to prevent discrimination. For example, everyone needs access to clean water, so it would be wrong to provide this for some people and not for others.[1]

However, if we applied this principle to health care, we would have to give the *same amount* of health resources to *everyone* regardless of need, eligibility or capacity to benefit. This doesn't sound plausible. Sick people need more care than healthy people. By contrast, if we distribute healthcare resources **unequally**, few people would accuse us of discriminating against the healthy. Healthy people do not normally make claims on resources they don't need.

If the goods are shared unequally, on what grounds will we do this? What sorts of things should we take into account in allocating resources? Different theories for resource allocation focus on different factors:

1. Getting **value for money** (economic evaluation) – decisions based around efficiency, cost-effectiveness or welfare maximisation.

2. Treating according to **need**.

3. Treating those who will **benefit** most.

4. Treating according to **desert** (not according to one's choice of pudding, but desert as in who is most deserving).

5. Upholding the **rights, autonomy and choice** of the individual patient.

6. Using **clinical** criteria to decide.

1. Getting value for money: cost effectiveness, efficiency and welfare maximisation.

Getting **value for money** is an important consideration in any system with limited resources. Obviously, interventions that are clinically effective should take priority over those that are useless. Ideally, all patients should be provided with the best treatments available. However, this cannot be done at any cost. As well as clinical effectiveness, we need to know if a treatment is **cost effective**. A procedure may work perfectly but cost the equivalent of a small yacht. To get the best value for money, we need to provide the greatest possible benefit within a fixed budget.

For Kevin the Consequentialist, the fairest way to distribute resources is to *maximise welfare*. As a utilitarian, Kevin may suggest using the concept of **Quality Adjusted Life Years,** or **QALYs.** This is the most commonly used example of a method known as cost-utility analysis.

QALYs are a way of numerically scoring the outcomes of treatments to help us compare the **overall benefits** of different treatment options.

How does the QALY system work?
* A year's life expectancy in **perfect health** is given a numerical value of 1.

* A year's life expectancy in **less-than-perfect health** is given a score of **less than 1**. How much less depends on how low we judge the patient's quality of life to be.

* Death is scored as 0.

* It is possible to judge a quality of life as being 'worse than death' by giving it a minus score.

The number given to a year's life expectancy in each state of health is thus **'quality adjusted'** according to how good the quality of life is judged to be.

QALYs allow us to judge treatments on both:

1. The increase in **length** of life produced.

2. The improvements in the **quality** of that life.

For example:
- An intervention providing an extra 10 years of life in perfect health would be worth 10 QALYs.

- An intervention improving someone's quality of life from 0.3 to 0.5 in a person with an expected 20 years to live would be worth (0.2 x 20) = 4 QALYs.

Once a particular treatment has been assigned a QALY value, it can be combined with information on the cost of the treatment. You can then calculate the **cost per QALY** and compare it with that of other treatments. The idea behind QALYs is that treatments with a **low cost per QALY** should be **prioritised.**

Examples of **QALY scores** given to common interventions (**cost per QALY**):

GP advice to stop smoking – £330
Hip replacement – £1500
Kidney transplant (cadaver) -£5900
Breast cancer screening – £6900
Hospital haemodialysis – £27 500

1983-4 prices corrected for inflation to 2004 values.[4]

QALYs are a straightforward approach to the problem of resource allocation, and have been widely used for a number of years. However, there are a number of **common criticisms** of QALYs:

a) **QALYs are ageist.** Treating younger people tends to produce a better QALY score, simply because younger people have a higher life expectancy. Therefore, they have more life years to gain than an older person receiving the same treatment. This position can be countered in a number of ways:

- This may be true for a one-off treatment, but what about treatments that need to be continued regularly for life? In this case the cost per QALY calculation might not necessarily favour the younger person, since the cost would rise the longer the patient lived.

- It can be argued that QALYs are not ageist as the actual age of patients is **not directly** taken into account. For example, take the case of an 80-year-old man who is expected to live for another 5 years following life-saving treatment. Under the QALY system, he would have the same priority for the treatment as a 40-year-old whose life-expectancy is also 5 years, because of some underlying, untreatable illness (assuming that both patients had a similar quality of life for those 5 years gained).[5]

- Indeed, some argue that QALYs are not ageist enough. In his **fair innings argument,** Lockwood argues that the 40-year-old should have *greater priority* than the 80-year-old.[6] This is because the 80-year-old has already had a 'fair innings'. He's benefited from 80 years of life, whereas his 'rival' has only enjoyed 40 years of life.

b) **QALYs discriminate against the disabled.** This is John Harris' 'double jeopardy' argument.[7] Disabled people are often judged to have a lower quality of life that able-bodied persons. Under the QALY system, they would appear to gain less benefit from a treatment than able-bodied individuals suffering from the same condition. Certain groups would thus be **doubly disadvantaged.**

c) **QALYs are not practical.** As many treatments do not yet have any QALY values, direct comparisons of the cost-effectiveness of treatments are often not possible.

d) **QALYs do not take account of need.** This is perhaps the most compelling argument for the inadequacy of QALY theory to solely resolve resource allocation problems. QALYs cannot be said to provide a 'fair' distribution of resources.

As we mentioned earlier, the fact that very ill people have greater medical need requires us to distribute resources *unequally* to meet this need. Aristotle's views on distributive justice were clear: treat equals equally, and **unequals unequally** in **proportion** to the **relevant inequalities** (this is known as the 'formal principle of equality').

The QALY based approach treats unequals **equally** as it ignores the differences in need for health care. It focuses only on the *benefits* of interventions. For distribution to be just, resources may need to be distributed to those in greatest need, even if the **QALY benefit** would be **lower** than treating a healthier group.

2. Needs theory

This states that some patients have a **special claim** to treatment because they have a **greater need** for it. One version of needs theory comes from John Rawls' work on distributive justice.[8] To explain his Needs theory, Rawls devised a thought experiment:

> Imagine that you are forced to choose between a number of hypothetical societies in which to live. Each society has a different way of distributing resources amongst its members. You have to make your choice from behind the '**veil of ignorance**'. In other words, you have no idea who you will be in that society. You could end up as a king or a beggar, beautiful or ugly, healthy or unhealthy.
>
> Rawls argued that *rational individuals* would 'play safe', and choose the society in which resources are distributed so that the **people who are worse off are better off than in any other system.** This is known as the 'difference principle'.

What are the implications of this in choosing between different **healthcare systems** (rather than societies in general)? How would we choose to allocate the scarce resources? If we accept Rawls' Needs theory, we would put **more resources** into those with the **worst health** to improve it as much as possible.

The main problems with this theory are:

a) Need is not the only criterion that should be taken into account. If it were, you would have to treat those who are the most badly off, **regardless of their ability to benefit** and future quality of life. Huge health resources would be used to produce marginal benefit for extremely sick people at the expense of other treatments and interventions.

For example, you might provide a heart transplant for an elderly man with heart failure rather than pay for statins for several hundred people with high cholesterol. Less serious but easily curable conditions such as ingrowing toenails would be ignored, leaving people suffering for marginal cost benefits. Preventative medicine would also be sidelined. We know that vaccination and the prevention of coronary heart disease are clinically and economically **more effective** than treating the resulting diseases. Deciding on the basis of need *alone* is therefore undesirable.

b) It is not clear that everyone would choose the 'difference principle' from behind the veil of ignorance. Some people might be prepared to gamble, hoping that they'll end up among the better off in society. However, Rawls also argued that as well as being the rational choice, the 'difference principle' was the **most just** option. Even if some people might not choose this hypothetical society themselves, it would still be the right choice for us to make on behalf of society as a whole.

To some extent, GMC guidance on prioritisation supports the policy of treating the neediest or sickest patients first:

'In determining priorities between individuals for a limited resource, clinicians should have regard for the three duties of care (to protect life and health, to respect autonomy and to treat justly). In many cases this assessment will give priority to the need to protect life and health, so that those whose **healthcare needs are greatest or most urgent** on clinical assessment will receive priority.'(emphasis added)[9]

Yet urgency is only one dimension of need. Under the current system, chronic conditions that cause considerable suffering may be marginalised in favour of conditions that need more immediate treatment. Satisfying the healthcare needs of both groups is desirable but logistically difficult.

Certainly, if we are to distribute resources **unequally** to patients on the basis of need, we need to be explicit about the **criteria used** to decide whether people are equal or unequal.

A further problem with the issue of need is: how do we differentiate between a legitimate need, and a desire or preference?[1] I 'need' a new desktop with more space and a DVD Rewriter, but how much of a need is it? And who should decide whether or not my need is legitimate? As this decision is based on values rather than facts alone, it raises problems when trying to ration objectively.

3. Ability to benefit

This principle prioritises patients most likely to benefit from treatment. It makes sense, after all, to use resources only where they will benefit patients. However, this theory would favour **treating curable illnesses,** even if minor, in preference to helping those with painful but incurable chronic conditions. It would also prioritise proven treatments over research and innovative therapies. This might slow down medical research and affect the health of future patients.

4. Desert

This controversial theory proposes that we allocate resources on the basis of a patient's *worth*. But how can we decide **who is most worthy of treatment?** Is it those who:

• have contributed the most to the health care system through taxes?

• do the most good in the local community?

• have not got self-inflicted illnesses?

• selflessly spend their days and nights writing textbooks for medics?

One possibility is to 'objectively' assess the **intrinsic worth** of the lives of potential patients. Imagine you have only one kidney for transplantation. You must choose one of two candidate patients:

> **Patient A: Veronica the Virtue Theorist's sister** – a 41-year-old widow and mother of 3 young children. A dedicated paediatric nurse, she also does voluntary work with the disabled, and is the sole carer for her elderly housebound mother.
>
> **Patient B: Adam Zapple's second cousin** – A 41-year-old heroin addict, currently serving a jail sentence for mugging an old lady. He has no family of his own, and has been unemployed all his life.

A consequentialist might choose patient A over patient B, on the basis that A produces more welfare in the world around her. If we let A die, she will leave three children as orphans. Her elderly mother will lose her sole carer and be transferred into residential care at considerable expense to the taxpayer. The local community will lose an excellent nurse and volunteer worker. If we let patient B die, it appears that few others will suffer greatly from his death.

Interestingly, surveys suggest that a significant proportion of the British public support considering factors such as a person's dependants when making such decisions.[10] However, there are compelling arguments against such a system:

* It is not the role of doctors to judge the social worth of patients.

* The provision of health care should not be used to reward people for their contribution to society.

* This would be impossible to judge in practice.

Some support the **ability to pay** as a legitimate consideration in deciding who should receive treatment. It can be argued that if the NHS will not fund a treatment, a patient should be allowed to pay for it himself. To some extent, this already happens through private practice. The ethics of private practice are complex, and there is no space to discuss them here. However, decision-making in resource allocation is not just a cost issue. Even if we increased the amount of money available for treatments, there will still be **other constraints** on the system, such as staff time or the number of organs for transplant.

Many people would support excluding those with a self-inflicted illness from treatment on the grounds of desert. This is discussed below.

5. Individual rights and patient autonomy

Do patients have any particular 'rights' to healthcare that may impact on decisions? Legally, all NHS decisions have to comply with the Human Rights Act 1998. The UK is also signed up to the International Covenant on Economic, Social and Cultural Rights. This gives its citizens the 'right to the highest attainable standard of physical and mental health'.[3] What this means in practice is not clear. Certainly, we could say that providing the 'highest attainable' standard of health to patients is unrealistic. The health system cannot provide such care to everyone all the time.

How much importance should we attribute to the patient's views on his medical care? The current government has supported the idea of 'patient choice', suggesting it could soon become a reality. Whether the rhetoric will be translated into practice remains to be seen. From an ethical perspective, patient choice appears desirable, as it would promote patient autonomy. Yet respecting the wishes of one patient may negatively affect the treatment of others. For example, what if a patient exercises his patient choice by demanding a more expensive treatment over a cheaper one? Accepting the request might have a knock-on effect on the medical care of other patients. One alternative would be to allow the patient to pay for the more expensive treatment. However, as mentioned earlier, cost is not the only constraint.

Medical/clinical criteria

Medical students are commonly presented with the ethical problem: one kidney, many desperately ill patients, who would you give the kidney to, and why? In practice, many people ignore the allocation theories given above. Surely, they argue, decisions should be made on the basis of *medical or clinical criteria alone*. This is a popular argument, probably because it seems to provide an easy answer. By relying on objective, medical criteria, it supposedly removes the difficult 'value-based' judgements about whom to treat. As Parker and Dickenson write, the *'use of medical criteria is often seen as a value-neutral "trump card" which puts paid to any further decisions about allocation of scarce health care resources'*. (p. 235)[11]

On reflection, we can see a number of **problems** with the sole use of clinical criteria. One problem is that the prognosis for many conditions is unpredictable. In addition, many of the factors that govern prognosis stem from the patient's social, educational and economic background. These factors also influence people's baseline level of health and their access to healthcare facilities. It is therefore **impossible to separate 'medical' factors** from other issues that affect healthcare.

As we have seen, all theories for resource allocation have problems. **No one theory alone is sufficient.** Questions of resource allocations are notoriously difficult. The important thing is to base the decisions on sound reasons and to make the reasoning process transparent.[3]

Decision-making in practice

No ethical theory alone can provide us with **satisfactory answers** on how to make rationing decisions in practice. So how can we make such decisions in a fair and reasonable way? Daniels and Sabin reviewed the ethical considerations of the various theories and developed an ethical approach to decision making, based on the *process* by which decisions are made. This is known as **accountability for reasonableness.**[12] It includes four criteria:

1. **Publicity:** The public should have *access* to decisions about resource allocation, and the rationales behind them.

2. **Reasonableness:** The rationales underlying decisions should appeal to *reasons and principles*.

3. **Appeals:** Decisions can be *challenged*.

4. **Enforcement:** *Regulation to* ensure that this actually happens.

In the UK, it is the Health Authorities (for hospital treatment) and Primary Care Trusts (for General Practice) who are responsible for making rationing decisions. Often, they will set up special committees or **priorities forums** to consider the relevant issues. In some areas, Clinical Ethics Committees are increasingly involved in the allocation process.

Many priorities forums are developing **ethical frameworks** to guide the decision-making process. One such framework (used in Oxfordshire) uses three main criteria to assess treatments.[13]

1. **Effectiveness** – the efficacy and value of each treatment should be considered, relative to the value of other treatments.

2. **Equity** – people in similar situations should be treated similarly. There should be no discrimination on the grounds of age, race, sex, family circumstances, lifestyle, learning disability, etc.

3. **Patient choice** – patients should be able to choose between treatments of similar efficacy.

It is important that Health Authorities and PCTs use such a **recognised framework** to make transparent and consistent decisions. The case below illustrates this need:

> **Case Example:** Three transsexuals, A, D and G, took North West Lancashire Health Authority to court for refusing to fund gender re-assignment surgery.
>
> The Health Authority had justified its decision by saying that it had a statutory obligation to care for all within its area with limited resources. This meant that some medical conditions were given lower priority.[14]

The Court of Appeal ruled that the Health Authority's decision-making policy was flawed, as it was not grounded in such a framework. The decision to decline the request for surgery was not necessarily wrong. It would have been lawful to refuse funding on the basis of prioritisation. However, the **way** the decision was made was unsatisfactory. In making its decision, the Health Authority should have:

• Accurately assessed the nature and seriousness of each type of illness.

• Determined the effectiveness of various forms of treatment for each condition.

• Given proper weight to that assessment in the formulation and individual application of its policy.[5]

As they had not treated transsexualism as an illness and failed to follow the above procedure, the decision was not considered just.

The impact of NICE

The National Institute for Clinical Excellent (NICE) was set up in 1999 to:

provide patients, health professionals and the public with authoritative, robust and reliable guidance on current 'best practice'.[15]

In giving recommendations for funding, NICE places much emphasis on the **evidence** for the **effectiveness** of treatments. In theory, the NHS should provide the treatments recommended by NICE. However, doctors still have the final decision on whether to provide treatment based on the patient's clinical circumstances.

At present, there is some debate over who is responsible for funding new treatments recommended by NICE. Should local organisations (Health Authorities and PCTs) find extra money out of their existing allocations? Should the Central Government provide more money? Either way, where will the extra money come from? The full impact of NICE recommendations is yet to be seen.

Case example: NICE have recommended that the NHS funds up to three cycles of IVF treatment for couples meeting specific criteria. Yet this guidance is not fully implemented at the present time. The Health Secretary said that, for the time being, couples will only be offered 1 cycle of IVF treatment. There is no *deadline* for full implementation of the guidance.[16]

How much responsibility should people take for their own health?

To what extent, if any, should we penalise those who damage their own health through their lifestyle choices? Should life-long smokers, for example, be entitled to treatments for self-induced lung disease, heart disease or gangrenous limbs. Some people would support withholding treatment from this group on the basis that:

1. The individual is **responsible** (at least in part) for bringing the problem on himself. Although aware of the risks, the person chose to smoke 20-a-day for the last 40 years.

2. As he is responsible for his plight, he is **less entitled** to health care than others who are ill through no fault of their own.[3] Why should the rest of us pay for someone else's bad habits? Is it fair that health-conscious citizens finance those who don't give a hoot about their health?

However, this position can be countered in several ways:

• **People's choices are not entirely free:** they are very much a product of their social circumstances. For example, poorer people are more likely to have poorer diets and to use alcohol, tobacco and drugs. Can we really blame people for obesity when market forces mean that calorie and fat-laden food is cheaper than healthier options? Genetic factors may affect the likelihood of individuals taking up health-damaging behaviours. Some argue that at least some heavy smokers and drinkers deserve sympathy rather than condemnation. Nicotine is an addictive drug which requires tremendous will power to give up. Similarly, alcoholism is an illness whose sufferers deserve support.

• **Complex disease aetiology:** the causal link between health damaging behaviour and disease is not always obvious. Adverse genetic interactions with environmental factors are beyond the control of the individual. There is also an element of bad luck. Only a percentage of heavy drinkers develop cirrhosis, for example, and we can't reliably predict who will.

- **Healthcare is so important that it cannot be compared** to other areas of life where we expect people to take responsibility.

- **Impractical and even counter-productive:** even if, in theory, we agree with the idea of discriminating against certain careless and blameworthy people, it would be *too difficult* to apply in practice. All aspects of life involve an element of risk. How much risk should be considered excessive? How restrictive will this be on people's autonomy? Should we refuse to treat the speeding driver injured in a car accident? The rugby player hit in the face by the ball? The cat owner with a piece of kitty claw imbedded in his cornea? How would the law deal with these questions, and what impact would it have on people and society?

> **Example:** Should we refuse to treat injured cyclists? Statistics show that cycling is a dangerous form of transport. But, by discouraging cycling, we may lead people to do less exercise. A more sedentary lifestyle may impact upon the rate of coronary heart disease and diabetes in the future.

What should the NHS fund?

Many people feel that the NHS should not fund cosmetic surgery, assisted reproduction, or 'lifestyle drugs' such as Viagra. Although some patients may desire these treatments, they are not essential for good health. But how do we decide what is 'essential to good health'? There is a subjective element to the decision. A significant proportion of the general public would give low priority to the funding of 'cosmetic' procedures, but what distinguishes 'cosmetic' from functional procedures is often unclear.[17]

A study investigating the reasons for, and the benefits of, breast reduction surgery illustrates this point.[17] The study was conducted to help the NHS decide whether it should fund such procedures in Oxfordshire. The women referred for the operation said that aesthetic concerns played only a small part in the reasons for undergoing surgery. Other physical, psychological or practical reasons were far more important. These patients had significantly lower scores on the SF-36 (a health rating scale) than the control group, showing that they had **significant physical and psychological morbidity** before surgery. This improved considerably after the procedure.

Similarly, the recent decision by NICE to fund a limited number of IVF cycles on the NHS recognises the considerable 'morbidity' that infertility can cause.[16] The 'need' for people to have their own biological children may differ from the need of a road accident victim for medical treatment, but it is still a need that requires attention. Many cases of infertility can now be treated at reasonable cost. If such a service produces considerable benefits for patients, we could argue that the NHS has good reason to fund it. No doubt those procedures at the 'boundaries of healthcare' will continue to generate much debate and controversy.

Summary

- Rationing is **inevitable** in our healthcare system.

- Ethical theories for the fair distribution of resources include:
  – Welfare maximisation
  – Needs Theory
  – Ability to benefit
  – Desert
  – Rights/Autonomy

- **No one theory is sufficient** to tell us what we should do.

- The **process** by which decisions are made is crucial. It needs to be reasoned, fair and transparent.

- Debate continues about which treatments should fall within the **remit** of the NHS, and how much **responsibility** people should take for their own health.

References

1. Schwartz L, Preece P, Hendry R. *Medical ethics:* a case-based approach. Philadelphia: Saunders, 2002.

2. Ashcroft, R. In vitro fertilisation for all? The question is for local purchasers to answer, not for NICE. BMJ 2003; 327: 511-2.

3. British Medical Association; Medical Ethics Today. London: BMJ Publishing Group, 2004.

4. Scambler G. *Sociology as applied to Medicine.* Fourth ed. Edinburgh: Saunders, 2000.

5. UK Clinical Ethics Network Website. URL: www.ethics-network.org.uk/Ethics/eresource.htm.

6. Lockwood M. Quality of life and resource allocation. In: Bell J, Mendus S, editors. *Philosophy and medical welfare.* Cambridge: Cambridge University Press, 1988.

7. Harris J. Double jeopardy and the veil of ignorance. *Journal of Medical Ethics* 1995;21:151-157.

8. Rawls J. *A Theory of Justice.* Cambridge, MA: Harvard University Press, 1971.

9. General Medical Council. Priorities and Choices. July 2000. URL: www.gmc-uk.org/standards/default.htm.

10. Hope T, Savulescu J, Hendrick J. *Medical ethics and law: the core curriculum.* Edinburgh: Churchill Livingstone, 2003.

11. Parker M, DIckenson D. *The Cambridge medical ethics workbook.* Cambridge: Cambridge University Press, 2001.

12. Daniels N. Accountability for reasonableness. *British Medical Journal* 2000;321:1300-1301.

13. Hope T, Hicks N, Reynolds D, Crisp R, Griffiths S. Rationing and the health authority. *British Medical Journal* 1998;317:1067-1069.

14. North West Lancashire Health Authority v. A, D and G, 2 FCR 525, 2000.

15. NICE website. URL: www.nice.org.uk.

16. NICE document CG11, Fertility: assessment and treatment for people with fertility problems. URL: www.nice.org.uk/pdf/CG011niceguideline.pdf.

17. Klassen A, Fitzpatrick R, Jenkinson C, Goodacre T. Should breast reduction surgery be rationed? A comparison of the health status of patients before and after treatment: postal questionnaire survey. *British Medical Journal* 1996;313:454-457.

Rights

We often hear of people having 'rights'. We hear of workers' rights, women's rights, social rights, human rights, children's rights and, of course, patients' rights. Patients, some say, have the right to healthcare. We hear that people have the right to liberty, and fetuses the right to life. Some people even talk of a right to be loved!

The study of rights falls within the field of legal and moral philosophy. It is a complex topic. In this section, we offer only a thumbnail sketch.

What is a right?

The definition of Geoffrey Marshall may be helpful:

'A right is a **form of entitlement arising out of moral, social, political or legal rules.**'[1]

It is useful to make a sharp distinction between legal rights and moral rights.

What is the difference between legal and moral rights?

A legal right is a **claim that gives rise to a remedy within a legal system.** The relevant government provides a structure both to deal with people who violate the legal rights of others and to compensate those whose rights have been infringed.

A moral right is a claim **on the behaviour of other people arising from social rules which are accepted by a community.** Unlike legal rights, however, **moral rights may not be enforced by law.** This does not mean that there is no sanction at all, but the sanction is social. When you violate a moral right, the sanction may range from an angry frown to social disapproval. No policeman will arrest you for violating a moral right.

A discussion of rights often generates confusion because the language of morals and the language of law are enmeshed. Laws are ultimately based on the moral principles of a society. Capital punishment, for example, is illegal in the European Union but permitted in the United States, Saudi Arabia, China and Japan. Underlying the law is a society's beliefs, and those beliefs can be seen as moral beliefs. History shows that some of these beliefs are not fixed. They evolve over time. Capital punishment has only been prohibited in the European Union since about 1981.

When lawyers argue about what the law is, they often refer to what is morally right. And when people invoke a moral right, they may also invoke the law as a source of morals. So, in everyday language, there is often a confusion between moral and legal rights. The two, however, are quite distinct, both conceptually and in practice.

A legal right can be **enforced by an authority,** which can be a court, a governmental agency or a policeman. If a person's legal right has been violated, he can thus seek a legal remedy. If there is no legal remedy, a lawyer would say that there is no corresponding legal right. **There cannot be a legal right without a remedy.** The enforcement of a moral right – to the extent that one can even speak of enforcement – is a much more ambiguous matter. If you promise to love me until death do us part and then fail to do so, what is my remedy? You may have violated a promise that I felt you were morally obliged to keep, but how do I enforce such a promise and what is my remedy for its violation?

Moral rights are thus far more slippery than legal rights. There are further problems with moral rights that do not exist for legal rights. We know where to find legal rights. They appear in statutes, regulations and reported cases decided by courts. We even know whom to ask to find out about them. A whole profession exists to advise us on our legal rights. But how do we find out about our moral rights? Where do we find them? Who decides what they are? Is there anyone we can ask for advice us on what they are? The answers to each of these questions has given rise to major philosophical theories which are beyond the scope of this introductory chapter.

Claim rights and liberty rights

When speaking of rights, a distinction is sometimes made between claim rights and liberty rights.

When we say someone has a right, we imply an entitlement. The right can **make another do certain things** (this is called a **claim** right), and it implies a corresponding duty on that person to respect it. So if I have a claim on Smith that he pay me £100, he has a corresponding duty to give me £100. Now, I can also have an entitlement that requires Smith **not to intervene** (this is a **liberty** right). If I want to read out this textbook at Hyde Park Corner, I can freely do so. I have a liberty right to read this textbook because there is a legal right to free speech. Smith cannot intervene to prevent me from exercising my liberty right. Yet my liberty right is not absolute. As Justice Holmes once remarked, not even the most stringent protection of free speech would allow a person to shout 'Fire!' in a crowded theatre!

Rights and duties

Imagine 'rights' on one side of the proverbial coin. On the other side are 'duties'. If you have a right not to be tortured, then others have a duty not to torture you (sounds plausible). If you claim to have a right to be loved, then others have a duty to love you (sounds implausible).

Duties can sometimes conflict, and people often invoke conflicting rights. If there is a decision-maker, such as a court or an ethics committee, then the court or committee must decide which right prevails. Consider the following scenario:

> *Adam Zapple, full of remorse, promises the recovering Debbie that he will visit her everyday for the next month. Three weeks later, on his way to his daily visit to the hospital, the only road leading to the hospital is inundated by animal rights activists shouting slogans against animal testing for drugs. He glances at his watch and realises that, unless he drives straight through the hordes of boisterous activists, he will not be allowed to visit Debbie. Visiting times are strict at the hospital. He briefly considers shutting his eyes and putting the pedal to the metal but, recalling all the advice from his 'stolen apple' episode, soon dismisses the idea.*

Since Adam Zapple made a promise to Debbie, he has a moral duty (arising from Debbie's claim right) to fulfil that promise but he also has a moral and legal duty not to kill the demonstrators (i.e. they have a right to life). If there is a conflict between the two rights, the weight of the latter clearly outweighs the duty to Debbie. As with the Four Principles, the agent must balance the weights of the competing rights in light of the situation at hand.

Thus the scope of Debbie's claim right does not extend to this particular situation. We sometimes speak of *prima facie* rights. We could then say that Debbie had a prima facie right to insist on Adam's visit and Adam had a prima facie duty to visit her, but on examination of all the circumstances we discover that Adam had a valid excuse for not performing his duty. Debbie, therefore, did not have an enforceable right, either legal or moral. A promise need not be upheld in certain circumstances. If I promise to buy you a copy of Hello magazine, you do not expect me to keep my promise if there is an earthquake or if I have been in a serious accident! There are limits to the scope of the right which may be tacit or implicit. There may be conditions which neither of the parties considered. It is thus not always easy to fix with certainty the scope of a legal or moral right until a specific case has arisen, and the difficult cases are usually those whose conditions neither party had anticipated.

Are moral rights absolute? Think of the right to life. Even a person's right to life can be infringed if that person is about to hack you to pieces with a razor-sharp machete! Self-defence may permit violating a person's right to life.

The duties arising from a moral right also need to be discussed. While you may have a right to life, do I have a moral duty to give you one of my kidneys if you lose one of yours? Surely not, although it can be argued that the state has a duty to provide you with medical treatment. Many books and articles in medical ethics try to argue that certain moral rights or duties exist, and the authors usually present elaborate arguments to explain why.

The philosophy known as **natural law** takes the position that certain moral rights are so fundamental that they cannot be outweighed. This is illustrated in the dialogue between Antigone and Creon, in Sophocles' play *Antigone*. King Creon had created a law forbidding the burial of Polyneices, Antigone's brother and the king's enemy. Antigone ignores the law and buries his brother. Creon arrests Antigone...

Creon: So you chose flagrantly to disobey my law?

Antigone: Naturally! Since Zeus never promulgated
              Such a law. Nor will you find
              That Justice publishes such laws to man below.
              I never thought your edicts had such force
              They nullified the laws of heaven, which
              Unwritten, not proclaimed, can boast
              A currency that everlastingly is valid,
              An origin beyond the birth of man.[2]

Other philosophies argue that moral rights arise out of a specific culture and that there are no universal moral rights. Yet it seems that all cultures share certain fundamental values, such as 'killing is wrong', but no culture takes the position that killing is always wrong. So the scope of a moral right is not always clear and may vary over time and from culture to culture.

Chapter 13

Medical ethics and human rights

In the field of medical ethics, both moral and legal rights are invoked. Think of the 'right to be told the truth', which is a moral right not always mandated by law, and the 'right to privacy', which is a legal right and a moral right. For a doctor to publish a patient's medical records would violate both the patient's legal and moral rights, but if the patient were to read a personal letter carelessly left behind by the doctor, he might be violating a moral duty but not a legal one. The term 'human rights', as used in the European Convention of Human Rights, are **rights based upon commonly accepted moral principles that have, by virtue of the treaty, become legal rights.**

Originating as fundamental moral rights derived from commonly shared values, they have been translated into legal rights. Failing to respect a human right protected by the European Convention can thus give rise to a legal remedy. In reality, as even the most cursory glance at today's newspapers will reveal, there are many parts of the world where human rights are violated without sanction. This is either because those rights have not been converted into legal rights or because, despite their conversion, the legal system is for one reason or another not enforcing them.

Moral rights have different weights and the decision-maker should perform a careful balancing act to arrive at a good decision. For legal rights, it is more accurate to talk of scope, rather than weight, since violating a legal right should, in theory, always result in sanction. Some human rights have universal scope. They apply in all circumstances. For example, according to the UN Declaration of Human Rights and the European Convention of Human Rights, it is wrong to torture someone irrespective of the circumstances. A consequentialist may well take issue with this absolutist claim. He might argue that if torturing a terrorist will reveal the location of a huge bomb in central London, then it is justified. That is not currently the law in the European Union. The scope of other human rights may be less clear. The right to 'respect for private and family life', which is relevant to medical confidentiality, does not mean that a doctor can never reveal anything. There are cases where the law requires a doctor to breach confidentiality (see chapter 4). In fact, the Convention itself recognises that the right has to be balanced against other considerations.

Many discussions in medical ethics allude to duties and obligations, but not specifically to rights. Despite the lack of explicit mention, human rights, either directly or indirectly, play an important role in contemporary debates in medical ethics. The BMA handbook on medical ethics and law expresses this well:

Many of the concepts that feature heavily in modern ethical analysis are either derived from statements of human rights or reflect them closely, but they are couched in term of moral rights and duties. (p. 5)[3]

Moral rights, legal rights, human rights, duties, obligations – you will see these terms in most of the current articles in medical ethics. Many of these articles will debate the existence, weight, and scope of these terms or try to apply them to a wide range of issues, from sex-selection to face transplants.

The Human Rights Act 1998 (adopted October 2000)

All the decisions of the NHS must be in line with the Human Rights Act 1998. This act states that all the rights included in the European Convention of Human Rights must be respected by public authorities in England. This includes, among others, the right to life, the right not to be tortured, the right to privacy, the right to travel, and the right to marry and found a family. The precise scope of each of these rights as they apply to medical practice in England is not always clear since the Act has only recently come into force. The scope of the rights will be clarified over time as new cases are decided by the courts, but the precise scope will never be *definitely* determined as new situations will arise constantly.

The Act requires doctors working in the NHS to respect the rights listed in the European Convention of Human Rights. Doctors will thus have to ask two questions when making decisions:

1. **Does this medical decision appear to violate a patient's right which is protected by the European Convention?"**

and

2. **Does my decision fall within the scope of the particular right?**

If the answer to both these questions is 'yes', the doctor cannot legally implement the decision unless there is a **legitimate competing legal interest** making it necessary in a democratic society to override the patient's prima facie rights.

Ask the expert: Professor Jonathan Montgomery, Professor of Health Care Law, University of Southampton

What is the likely impact of the Human Rights Act on doctors in the UK?

The Human Rights Act 1998 has **immense potential to change the shape of medical law in the UK. Decisions around dying** need to take into account not only the right to life (Article 2 of the European Convention on Human Rights) but also Article 3 (protection from inhuman and degrading treatment). Those same articles may also be relevant to **resource allocation decisions**, particularly when considered in the light of the prohibition of discrimination in relation to human rights under Article 14. Article 8 of the Convention, **respect for private and family life,** goes to the heart of the position in which patients find themselves. It is this article that protects autonomy and privacy. Although the early case law using the Human Rights Act showed some judicial timidity in reviewing established principles, this picture may be beginning to change. At present, the use of the **Bolam test** to govern even decisions about withdrawing life prolonging treatment (i.e. the Bland decisions) has been held as **compatible with human rights** (NHS Trust v M; NHS Trust v H [2001] 2 FLR 367). The courts have also **rejected attempts to use the Human Rights Act as a basis for a right to treatment** (R v NW Lancashire HA, ex p A [2000] 1 FCR 525). However, there is a **growing interest in autonomy claims under article 8,** including the right to request treatment as well as refuse it, which suggests that the judges may be looking to support a more active role for patients and permit less control to health professionals over their work than has traditionally been allowed (e.g. R (Burke) v GMC [2004] EWHC 1879). More decisions will need to be brought to court following the ruling of the European Court of Human Rights in Glass v UK [2004] 1 FLR 1019 that it was improper of a hospital to decide to withhold resuscitation and impose pain relief against parental wishes unless there was either an emergency or a referral to a judge. In short, there seems to be a **move towards closer regulation through law** than was prevalent prior to the implementation of the Human Rights Act. It has taken a little time for this impact to be felt, but it is likely to become increasingly significant.

Summary

- A right is a **form of entitlement** arising out of moral, social, political or legal rules.

- There is a **sharp distinction** between legal and moral rights.

- Legal rights necessarily give rise to a **remedy within a legal system.** Moral rights may not be enforced by law, but often have **social sanctions.**

- There is a distinction between **claim rights,** which make other people do certain things, and **liberty rights,** which prevent people from intervening.

- **Rights** give rise to **duties.**

- Both moral and legal rights are invoked in medical ethics.

- All decisions of the NHS must follow to the **Human Rights Act 1998.** Doctors will have to respect the rights listed in the European Convention of Human Rights.

- The impact of the Human Rights Act in the UK will be increasingly significant.

References

1. Marshall G. Rights, options and entitlements. In: Simpson A, editor. *Oxford Essays in Jurisprudence*. Oxford: Clarendon Press, 1973.

2. Sokol R. Was Antigone right? *Justice after Darwin*. Charlottesville, Virginia: Michie, 1975:24-25.

3. *Medical Ethics Today; British Medical Association*. Second edition ed. London: BMJ Publishing Company, 2004.

Passing medical ethics exams

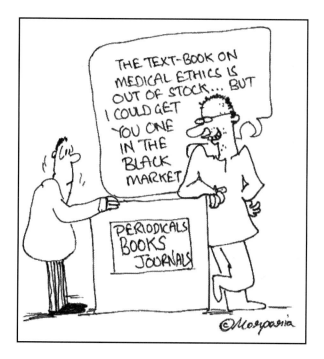

You should, by now, have all the factual knowledge you need to pass your medical ethics exams. But knowledge, alas, is not enough! It must be applied properly. As Osler said [*Kevin the consequentialist grabs his handy pillow*]:

A student may know all about the bones of the wrist, in fact he may carry a set in his pocket and know every facet and knob and nodule in them, he may have dissected a score of arms, and yet when he is called to see Mrs. Jones who has fallen on the ice and broken her wrist, he may not know a Colles' from a Potts' fracture, and as for setting it *secundum artem* [by the rules of art], he may not have the faintest notion, never having seen a case.[1]

The same is true of medical ethics. All the information in this book is useless if you don't apply it to your own experience on the wards or to your medical ethics exams. To remedy this lack of practical application and avoid the pitfalls of ignorance, we have asked teachers and examiners of medical ethics in the United Kingdom what they love and hate about typical student answers in exams. All of them teach medical students, set questions and mark exam scripts. Their pearls of wisdom should ensure that you improve your exam technique, get rid of your bad habits, and focus on what examiners are looking for. We have tried to cover all the different types of exam styles used by British medical schools, from short answer questions to long essays to OSCEs.

Answering a medical ethics exam question is quite different from answering questions in surgery or anatomy. Although some answers in medical ethics are either right or wrong, many are good or bad, rather than undeniably right or wrong. Examiners occasionally want you to 'use your nut' and that is precisely what you should do!

Things examiners love and hate

Dr Richard Ashcroft, Reader in Medical Ethics, Imperial College, London.

LOVE

- **A clear, well-stated conclusion.**

- A balanced presentation of the arguments **for and against** the conclusion.

- An accurate statement of the **legal position** (where relevant).

- Sensitivity to the **psychological, social and cultural dimensions** of the patients' and doctors' experiences.

- A **clearly set out, reasoned and valid argument** from accurately stated premises to the conclusion the candidate is defending.

HATE

- **Lists.**

- 'On the one hand, on the other' – **dithering** without making up your mind!

- **'In my opinion...'** – I am not interested in your opinion, I am interested in whether you are right!

- **Poor spelling** (especially of key technical terms) and **bad grammar.**

- **Misciting** legal cases and Acts of Parliament (e.g. when you cannot remember the right case, citing the wrong one 'just in case', or getting the name and date of the Act wrong).

How to pass

- Go to lectures.

- Read the literature.

- Discuss the topics with your colleagues.

- Prepare properly for the exam (revise, look at past papers or questions, test your own knowledge and understanding).

- Get the basics right first, and then set out the detail and the nuances of the argument.

Chris Cowley, Lecturer in Medical Ethics, University of East Anglia Medical School.

LOVE

- Explicit attempts to **define key ethical concepts,** especially in borderline cases.

- An attempt to **use a detailed example** to focus the answer.

- The use of **ordinary moral concepts** rather than the technical jargon from the medical ethics literature.

- An awareness of where a given illness and treatment will fit into the patient's particular on-going life; an awareness of the multiple meanings of the body and the person (i.e. an awareness that the body is not a machine to be merely fixed or a puzzle to be solved).

- A persistent attempt to **describe two** (or more) **sides of a debate,** while taking rigorous care to do justice to both the complexity of the issues and to the intelligence of the respective proponents.

HATE

- **Regurgitation** of any of the 'Four Principles' as if this alone somehow answered the question: 'We shouldn't do X because of the principle of non-maleficence.' Of course, we shouldn't harm the patient, but you haven't told me what 'harm' constitutes in this case!

- Too great a **reliance on the concept of rights,** coupled with an assumption that this answers the question: 'We shouldn't do X because it would violate the patient's human rights.' Which right? Can that right ever be overridden when, for example, the patient's life is at stake? When other patients' lives are at stake? Rights always give the impression of arbitrary stipulation.

- Too great a **reliance on simplistic utilitarianism (i.e. maximise welfare)** as the guiding principle to resource allocation, without giving sufficient weight to the uncertainties involved in measurement and comparison, to the place of justice and desert, and to the patient's own perspective.

- Too quick and too glib a descent into a **facile relativism:** 'there are no right and wrong answers in ethics'. Of course there are! Slavery is absolutely wrong, for example. 'It's all subjective and personal' – try telling that to a victim of obvious injustice. The main point here is: whatever you may say, none of us behave as if we were subjectivists about ethics.

- Using expressions such 'research has shown' or 'evidence suggests' with no awareness of how irrelevant research and evidence are to many ethical questions.

Additional tips

- What is important in ethics is **cultivating a particular type of attitude and sensitivity** over the longer term.

- Read the question carefully, make sure you **answer it explicitly** rather than taking it as a cue to regurgitate. If you have to go on a diversion, tell the reader why this is necessary to answer the question.

- Ethics has to be about a *problem,* so the first job in any answer is to **make the problem plausibly clear,** e.g. the two sides of the argument, the disagreement over the relevant definitions and descriptions. An answer to an ethics question could also include consideration of a simplistic answer to the problem and a discussion of why such an answer fails.

Dr Piers Benn, Lecturer in Medical Ethics and Law, Imperial College, London.

- Be **relevant.**

- **Read the questions** – can't be repeated enough!

- Try to **deal with counterarguments** to your own position. Listing arguments will probably do for short-answer questions but some critical input is always a bonus.

- Ethics is usually taught alongside basic law and some students fail because they just **haven't grasped the law** and make all kinds of confusions. Some students, for example, still think that respecting refusal of life-saving treatment amounts to assisted suicide.

Dr Mike Parker, Professor of Bioethics, University of Oxford.

Tips on answering medical ethics essay questions

- A medical ethics essay should **present an argument**. That is, it should pose a question (or respond to the one set), list the possible courses of action and give reasons for and against those options, come to a conclusion and say why one set of reasons was more convincing than the others. **An essay should not be descriptive** e.g. 'X says this, Y says this and the GMC says the other'.

- A case-based medical ethics essay **should identify the ethical problem**. What is it about this case that is ethically difficult as opposed to practically or clinically difficult? What ethical problems does it pose? Often bad essays are bad because they don't start with a case that presents a moral problem.

- Similarly, essays sometimes start with a case that does present an ethical problem but then go on to 'resolve' the case **without giving moral arguments,** e.g. 'I think in a case like this the doctor should have accepted the son's view about his mother's best interests and withheld treatment', but why?

To be avoided:

- Essays that don't make a distinction between what the law says, what the guidelines say, and what is morally the right thing to do.

- Essays that don't recognise that **key terms** used in the guidelines and in clinical practice **require value judgements and are not unproblematic** e.g. 'best interests', 'quality-of-life', 'serious harm', 'futile' and so on.

Dr Nafsika Athanassoulis, Lecturer in Medical Ethics, University of Leeds Medical School.

LOVE

- **Clarity** – the reader should be able to easily understand what you want to say and the *implications of your arguments.*

- **Structure** – the assignment should have a beginning, a middle and an end. It should have an aim and clearly show how this *aim* will be achieved.

- **Critical thinking** – the assignment should *critically engage with ideas,* raise objections and try to formulate replies.

- **Relevance** – the assignment should *answer the question and make reference to relevant pieces of literature.* This includes good *integration between clinical and philosophical ideas.*

- **Originality** – for extra points, surprise me with something new!

HATE

- **Too descriptive** – a catalogue of other people's ideas with no effort to critically assess them.

- **Irrelevant** – *off the topic,* not answering the question.

- **Confused** – *muddled* about philosophical ideas, concepts and theories and how they relate to each other. *Factual mistakes and misinterpretations,* as well as misunderstandings of arguments. Includes poor structure, uncertainty about what the assignment is trying to argue for or how it will do so.

- **Too general** – a broad discussion of *everything vaguely relevant* to the topic. Lacking in focus and in-depth analysis.

- **Anything but ethics** – legal and clinical points are certainly relevant to an ethical discussion, but *exclusive, often descriptive discussions of the law or basic science are not philosophy.*

Tips on giving medical ethics presentations

- Try to **speak to the audience** rather than read a full text.

- Talk in a **relaxed manner**, thinking about what you are saying as you are saying it and trying to explain the ideas you know to your audience, rather than trying to remember a memorised speech.

- **Do use overhead projectors and PowerPoint,** but don't be limited by them. If you have a better idea, use it! You can stage debates, role-play a case study, video-tape an interview (get patient consent or possibly Research Ethics Committee approval beforehand though!), conduct a mini-study...**use your imagination.**

- **Interact with your audience.** Ask them to think about a question, perform a task, confer with each other, etc.

- **Time yourself** and stick to your time. An audience gets tired easily, never go over the allocated time. If necessary, omit details (make them available on a handout or electronically) in favour of keeping to the time. Make a few points clearly and repeat them often, rather than lots of rushed points.

Making use of the Four Principles

To refresh your memory, the Four Principles are:

1. Respect for autonomy
2. Beneficence
3. Non-maleficence
4. Justice

The Four Principles, by themselves, do not tell us much that we do not already know. It is pretty obvious that we should do good to others, avoid causing them harm, respect their autonomy, and treat people fairly. To be of any use, they need to be expanded and applied in a particular context. Like all moral theories, the Four Principles can be used with insightful virtuosity or, more often than not, massacred by empty mentions of their name alone (e.g. 'do this because of the principle of the beneficence'). The Four Principles approach requires you to think carefully about various aspects of the case at hand. You cannot simply apply the principles like a mathematical formula, hoping that you will arrive at the required answer.

There are two main areas of debate when applying the Four Principles:

1. The **scope** of the principles, i.e. to whom do the principles apply?
2. What to do when principles **conflict** with each other.

Scope

We already encountered questions of scope in the previous chapters, most notably: do we have an obligation towards fetuses? Does the scope of the principles of beneficence and non-maleficence include fetuses? Should we respect the autonomy of competent children?

The principle of respect for autonomy should apply to all autonomous agents, but what constitutes an autonomous agent? Our answer to that question will affect the scope of the principle's application. So, if X is an autonomous agent, we have a *prima facie* duty to respect his autonomy. But if X is *not* autonomous, we don't owe him this obligation. The difficulty lies in deciding whether X is sufficiently autonomous to fall within the scope of the principle.

The principle of justice requires us to allocate our resources fairly, but to whom? To our friends, our community, our country, the world, all future people? We saw in the previous chapter that persons possess various rights, such as the right to life. But, again, who is entitled to such a right? Both you and I have a right to life, but what about the plant on my desk or the bird outside? What about cats, dogs and chimpanzees? What about fetuses and patients in a permanent vegetative state?

Although the principles of beneficence and non-maleficence go hand in hand in the clinical context, there is a clear difference in scope between the two. Raanan Gillon uses the following scenario to illustrate this point: imagine walking down the road and seeing a beggar holding a small tray. Few would say that you have a moral obligation to give the beggar some money, but everyone would agree that you have an obligation not to kick him in the teeth! In short, the scope of the principle of non-maleficence is *far greater* than the scope of the principle of beneficence. In normal circumstances, we have obligations of beneficence to *only a few people* but obligations of non-maleficence to *everyone*. In medicine, the scope of the duty of beneficence is partially established: doctors and nurses have a duty of beneficence to their patients, by virtue of their special relationship.[2]

Conflict

In difficult ethical situations, two or more of the *prima facie* principles will conflict. To resolve the conflict, you will have to give weights to each of the principles (this will depend on the specific circumstances) and, by balancing the weights, determine which principle should take priority.

Deriving rules and 'specifying'

In chapter 2, we saw how the principle of respect for autonomy requires doctors to do certain things:

* Obtain informed consent

* Keep patients' secrets

* Avoid deception

* Help patients make decisions

* Communicate effectively

These rules were **derived** from the principle. You will have noticed that rules are **more specific** than principles. Similar rules can be derived by 'specifying' the other principles.

What is specification?

Specification is '**filling in**' principles to give them content that will be useful in solving ethical problems. This may involve deriving rules from them (such as 'do not lie') or adding more specific clauses to the rules. Deciding on the scope of the principles is a form of specification.

Why specify?

On their own, principles are too abstract to provide a guide to action. They need to be given more content. Take, for example, the principle to avoid harm. Behind the apparent simplicity of the principle lies all kinds of further questions: What counts as harm? Who should judge this? Does violating a person's right harm him? Can you harm someone if he is unaware of it? Specifying principles by modifying or expanding their content can make them relevant to new ethical problems and contexts. Specification allows principles to **adapt** to individual cases, and helps to **resolve conflicts** between the principles.

> **Example of specification**
>
> A doctor has a patient who needs a kidney. Vaguely remembering the principle of beneficence, which obliges him to provide net benefit to his patient, he decides to illegally (but very cheaply) buy one from a poor, non-English speaking Bangladeshi peasant over the Internet and gives it to his patient. This is clearly undesirable, so, in light of such a case, we should specify the principle of beneficence by adding '...provide net benefit *using means that are both legally and morally permissible*'.

It is important, when you specify a principle, that you can **justify** why you added that content. You cannot just specify without giving a reason. Note also that, unfortunately, specifying principles does not always resolve conflicts between different principles! In such cases, you will have to balance the conflicting principles and pick the weightier one.

Balancing Principles: Along with specification, you should **balance** the moral norms derived from the principles. When you come to a decision, you should give good reasons why you think one moral norm (for example, 'keep promises') should outweigh another ('do not lie').

If a hundred people were asked to analyse a medical ethics case using the Four Principles approach, some people may well reach different conclusions. Beauchamp and Childress have compiled a list of reasons why people can disagree about moral matters.(p. 21)[3] The reasons include:

1. They don't agree on the **facts** (e.g. Kevin might think that an act will cause X amount of suffering but Dan thinks that it will cause far more).

2. They disagree about the **scope** of the moral norm (e.g. does the obligation not to kill innocent humans include fetuses?).

3. They **disagree about the relevant norms** (e.g. is there a duty to disclose all relevant information about a patient's illness?).

4. They **disagree about how to specify** the norms.

5. They **disagree about how much weight** each norm should have in the circumstances.

6. There is a **genuine moral dilemma** (i.e. you should do X *and* you should do Y, but you cannot do both!).

7. There is not enough information or evidence to reach an agreement.

Disagreement does not, in itself, mean that we should just give up. There may be good reasons for disagreeing, as well as terrible reasons. If the reasons are bad, we should try to point out what is wrong about them. If the reasons are good, then we can just agree to disagree and find a compromise.

Applying the Four Principles to real medical ethics problems

On their own, then, the principles do not resolve moral conflict. However, they can help us to identify moral problems and to generate good reasons for choosing a particular course of action. The Four Principles approach can be used as a **diagnostic tool** – an ethical stethoscope – to discern the ethical rumblings and murmurs embedded in a case. Consider the case of Mrs B (see box below), a real and thorny case which one of us encountered when working as a clinical ethicist a few years ago.

The case of Mrs B

History:

- Mrs B, a 29-year-old female, arrives in the Intensive Care Unit with severe meningitis. She is 23 weeks pregnant.

- She falls into a coma, and then into a persistent vegetative state. She is intubated and ventilated.

- Tests reveal that Mrs B is HIV positive. The result is communicated to her husband, who is greatly distressed by the news.

- The unborn baby has a 30-40% chance of being infected with HIV.

- The husband is consulted about what to do, but asks the advice of the healthcare team.

Should Mrs B be kept alive? What are the ethical difficulties in this case?

Important: When analysing a case, the first step is to **gather as much information about the case as possible.** A single fact can change the outcome of an ethical analysis! Most of the time, you will just have to make do with what you are given.

The second step is **identifying the ethical problems** in the case. This is where the Four Principles come in handy.

Let us go through the Four Principles and see what ethical difficulties we can find. This is not a comprehensive analysis of the case, but merely an exercise to show that the Four Principles can flag up the ethical issues of even the most complex cases.

Principles of Beneficence and Non-Maleficence

Doctors need to act in the best interests of a) the mother and b) the fetus. Let us consider each in turn:

- **Is it in Mrs B's best interests to be kept alive?**

To answer this, imagine if Mrs B had not been pregnant, but merely in a PVS state. This ensures that we focus only on Mrs B's best interests. What would decide then?

The degree of cognitive function is important is deciding what is in Mrs B's best interests. Can she feel pain? Is she sufficiently aware to have interests? Is there any chance of recovery, however partial? If so, what are the chances? These are all empirical questions, but they are clearly relevant to the ethical problem.

Perhaps we can say that it is not against her interests to be kept alive, since she presumably has no cognitive capacity.

• **Is it in the best interests of the fetus for Mrs B to be kept alive?**
There are main two options here:

YES, it is better to be born with no mother and with HIV than not to be born at all (this is the worst case scenario, as the baby has only a 30-40% chance of being infected with the virus).

NO, it is better *not* to be born at all than to be motherless and HIV positive.

Whatever option you prefer, make sure you back it up with good arguments.

You might want to argue that the unborn baby *currently* has no interests, since he is only 23 weeks old. You can say that, this early in the pregnancy, the duties deriving from the principles do not apply to the fetus (i.e. it is out of the principles' scope). Again, this is a contentious claim so make sure you expand on the argument.

Possible conflict: Assuming that it is against the best interests of the mother to be kept alive but in the fetus' best interests for the mother to carry on living, we have a conflict between our duty of beneficence towards the mother and the duty of beneficence/non-maleficence towards her fetus (if we accept that the fetus lies within the scope of the relevant principles).

Note: In the UK, remember that a fetus has **no legal status until birth**. The legal obligations of the doctors are therefore to the mother. Remember also that law and ethics do not always map neatly onto each other. In this case, you may think that there is a potential conflict between a doctor's legal and moral duties. This may be worth mentioning in your answer!

Principle of Respect for Autonomy

Let us go through some of the people involved in the case:

- **Autonomy of Mrs B** – as Mrs B is in PVS, she is not *currently* autonomous. But has she left an advance directive? Does she have a next of kin or relatives that could inform the medical team of what she *would have* wanted in this situation? At the very least, the relatives could give some indication of her values and beliefs. Her husband could theoretically provide valuable information, but he is so traumatised by the situation that he hands over the decision to the medical team. There is no advance directive, and no other way of knowing what she would have wanted. One option would be to wait for the husband to recover from the initial shock, but time is of the essence since the pregnancy is progressing!

- **Autonomy of the fetus** – the fetus is not currently autonomous. It therefore falls outside the scope of the principle of respect for autonomy. 'Pro-life' advocates could use all kinds of arguments here to support a moral obligation to keep the fetus alive. See the chapter on Human Reproduction for details (chapter 6).

- **Autonomy of the husband** (next of kin) – the husband delegated the decision to the healthcare team. This is not inconsistent with respect for autonomy, of course, as long as the **choice to delegate** was autonomous.

Note: in an exam, you might want to spend some time on the concept of autonomy (e.g. what is it? What does it require? why is it important?).

Principle of Justice

Justice as the 'fair allocation of scarce resources' (this concerns 'distributive justice').

- If Mrs B is kept alive, she has a high probability of breathing unassisted. This will entail many years of palliative and supportive care. This is extremely costly and will inevitably divert considerable sums of money away from areas where they might be urgently needed.

This raises the question: does the patient's interests always come first?

Possible Conflict: If you believe that that it is in the best interests of the mother and/or fetus to be kept alive, then there may be a conflict between the principle of beneficence, which gives you an obligation to care for your patient(s), and the principle of justice, which gives you an obligation to society. But what are the limits of these obligations? Does a doctor have a duty to benefit his patient *at all costs*, even if that means endangering his own life? (think of a doctor treating a patient infected with a virulent strain of the Ebola virus!). Is it morally acceptable to spend an enormous amount of money to support one PVS patient who has virtually no chance of regaining consciousness, when that money could be used more fruitfully elsewhere (e.g. buying more dialysis machines)? Here you may want to invoke some ethical theories, such as consequentialism and deontology, to enrich your answer. You may also want to highlight their respective advantages and disadvantages (see chapter 1).

Finally, in light of your analysis, you will need to look at the possible choices and **to recommend an action plan**. What is your decision on this ethical case, and what reasons can you give for *and against* your decision? Don't be worried about voicing your personal opinion; just make sure you back it up with sound arguments.

The case of Mrs B is an incredibly rich case, and you may well find further ethical questions which we neglected. Nevertheless, our brief analysis of the case has shown that the Four Principles can provide a useful tool with which to untangle the many ethical threads in a medical ethics case. They do not give you a neat solution to the problems, but they ensure that you do not miss any of the major ethical issues. When applied correctly, they clarify the ethical dimension of a case by flagging up key issues, raising important questions and stimulating thought.

The Seven Steps to Ethical Decision-Making in Practice

1. Gather all the relevant facts about the case at hand.
2. Recognise that there is an ethical problem in the case.
3. Find out what the ethical problems are (you may want to use the Four Principles approach to help you).
4. List all the possible options available.
5. Make a reasoned, informed decision on which option to adopt.
6. If possible and appropriate, run your decision and reasoning with trusted colleagues.
7. If satisfied, implement decision. If not, think again.

Examples of exam questions

Below is a typical short answer question used in the Imperial College Medical Ethics and Law exams. These questions test your knowledge of basic law and ethics.

Peter Smith is 17 years old. He has just had a motorcycle accident, and been admitted to A & E. In the course of his accident, he has sustained a number of injuries, including a badly broken leg, and he is bleeding heavily. When you see him, he is still conscious, but seems to be losing consciousness due to shock and loss of blood. You tell him that he needs an emergency operation. He says "no blood, no blood!" before passing out. You notice that he has in his wallet an advance directive stating that he is a Jehovah's Witness and refuses to have a blood transfusion, even if this would save his life.

a) What are the legal conditions under which a person under the age of 18 can consent to medical treatment? (4 marks)

Answers, with marking scheme: Children who are **16 or 17 are presumed competent to consent** (under the Family Law Reform Act 1969) (1 mark), and so **can consent unless deemed mentally incompetent** for some other reason, such as loss of consciousness or serious mental illness (1 mark). Children *under 16* can only consent if they are found to be **Gillick competent** (1mark). A child is Gillick competent if he or she has **sufficient understanding and maturity to understand fully what is proposed** (1 mark).

b) Should children's refusal of life-sustaining treatment be respected? Give two ethical arguments for and two against respecting minors' wishes (4 marks).

Answers:

Reasons for: 1. if a child is legally able to consent to treatment, then **logically he or she is also able to refuse it** (1 mark). 2. Respecting the decisions of mature children is the **best way to respect their autonomy** and human dignity (1 mark).

Reasons against: 1. Children are usually **not the best judges of what is in their own best interests** (1 mark). 2. The aim of medical and parental care of children is to raise them to sufficient maturity so that they can make their own decisions, but until that time, **we may need to override their wishes in their best interests** (1 mark).

Note: there are other possible answers here!

c) What are the conditions necessary for an advance directive to be legally binding?

Answer: An advance directive should have been **signed by someone who is competent to make the decision** at the time of writing (1 mark). It must be **specific and applicable to the circumstances** now applying (1 mark). It must also have been **signed by someone who understands the consequences of refusing treatment and the available alternatives to treatment** (1 mark). It should also be clear that the patient **has not competently changed their mind** since signing the advance directive (1 mark).

d) Suppose Peter's mother arrived and insisted that her son not be given a blood transfusion. Should you comply? Give both legal and ethical reasons for your answer (3 marks).

Answer: Legally, doctors **do not have to accept a parental refusal** regarding life-saving treatment, and have a **duty to act in the child's best interests** (2 marks). Ethically, we may have a **duty to protect minors from parental abuse and neglect** (1 mark). [We could also argue that we should respect the mother's wishes as we must act in Peter's *general* best interests, not just his medical best interests, and membership of a community may be very important to him (this would also get 1 mark)].

Passing the medical ethics OSCE
(Objective Structured Clinical Examination)

Some medical schools have a medical ethics station at the OSCE. It is not difficult, but you will need to think on your feet. To impress the examiners, you will need to:

- Identify the main issues of each scenario, and define any ethical concepts.

- Discuss the concepts and issues relevant to the scenario.

- Show an awareness and understanding of the feelings and ethical issues experienced by the individuals concerned.

- Suggest ways of approaching the situation, appropriate to the case scenario or material presented, including the recognition of a compromise solution.

- Show an awareness of the pros and cons of your approach, including its possible consequences.

As always when you read the requirements for a test, it sounds harder than it is. After all, you cannot go into much depth in the 5 to 10 minutes you have at the station.

Dos and Don'ts for Medical Ethics OSCEs

Dr Martin von Fragstein, Lecturer in General Practice, University of Nottingham.

Do:
- Remain focused.

- Identify the issues/problems presented.

- Reflect on the differing perspectives either from an ethical perspective or directly relating them to the individuals involved.

- Be able to clearly define key concepts and/or principles.

- Reflect on the feelings that might be generated.

- Acknowledge the limits of your knowledge.

- Stick to the time limit.

Don't:
- Waffle.

- Repeat the story – you may be sitting in front of the person who wrote the paper!

- Guess at material you don't know.

- Get side-tracked onto one small part.

Here is an actual OSCE scenario with a marking scheme kindly provided by the medical school in question.

Scenario

A 57-year-old lady is dying of breast cancer and wishes to know the extent of her illness. You know that she has extensive metastases. Her condition deteriorates and she is pleading with you to make her comfortable (not kill her). She is pain free and terminal agitation is causing her some distress. However the husband very quickly says "but we don't want anything to sedate her".

Things to mention

1. Respect for autonomy
2. Right to refuse treatment
3. Access to health care of her choice
4. Distinction between killing and letting die
5. Pain management
6. Family issues

Marking scheme

Excellent = mention 4 or more issues
Good = mention 3 issues
Satisfactory = mention 2 issues
Fail = mention 1 issue

Factors affecting the situation

1. Ethical principles applied in scenario (beneficence, autonomy, non-maleficence)
2. Experience of past health care
3. Health beliefs (religious or social)
4. Human rights issues
5. Medical management

Marking scheme

Excellent = presents a clear, balanced argument of all the issues and is able to reflect on the potential dilemmas. Factually correct.

Good = discusses most of the issues with some ability to reflect on the balance of arguments. Gets most facts correct.

Satisfactory = basic understanding of a few issues. Is aware that arguments are present on both sides. Based on minimum key facts.

Fail = unable to argue any issues coherently and unable to see balance of arguments. Unable to present any key facts.

Presentation of potential solutions, relevant principles and feelings of individuals involved

1. Use of communication skills
2. Autonomy
3. Beneficence
4. Justice
5. Non-maleficence
6. Consent (competency)
7. Denial
8. Anger

Marking scheme

Excellent = able to present clear strategies for the situation and potential compromise. Understands clearly all relevant ethical and legal principles. Can identify feelings generated.

Good = presents some strategies to deal with the situation. Understands most of the ethical and legal principles. Identifies some feelings generated.

Satisfactory = presents a few strategies to deal with situation. Understands at least 2 principles fully. Recognises feelings may exist.

Fail = only able to identify one strategy (or less!). Does not understand any principles (one is not enough). Unable to recognise any feelings.

Overall assessment of presentation

1. Prompting
2. Fluency
3. Empathy

Marking scheme

Excellent = arguments and information presented with no prompting. Clear balance of argument. Appears empathic/sympathetic to the dilemma.

Good = some prompting needed. Balanced argument with minimal hesitation. Mostly uses language indicating empathy.

Satisfactory = information prompted for and presents an argument with some hesitation and structure. Uses language with some empathy.

Fail = requires a lot of prompting. Unable to order argument. No evidence of empathy.

Summary

Medical ethics exams are different to other medical exams. They test knowledge as well as critical thinking. Regurgitating material will probably get you through them, but, to do well, you will need to apply your knowledge based on the case at hand. For short answers, you should demonstrate that you know the basics. You should understand the basic idea behind the ethical principles and know the relevant law. For longer answers, you should demonstrate the complexity of the subject matter, presenting various sides of the argument before arguing persuasively for your position. For OSCEs, you should identify and understand the main issues and suggest ways to tackle them in a compassionate manner. We believe the Four Principles approach can provide a useful starting point for the analysis of medical ethics cases. Applying the Four Principles, dissecting cases into their ethical components and arguing convincingly for your position are skills acquired through practice. In preparation for your exams, it is therefore essential that you look over past papers and practise answering questions under timed conditions.

References

1. Verney R, editor. *The student life; the philosophy of Sir William Osler.* Edinburgh: E & S Livingstone Ltd, 1957.

2. Gillon R. Medical ethics: four principles plus attention to scope. *British Medical Journal* 1994;309:184-188.

3. Beauchamp T, Childress J. *Principles of Biomedical Ethics.* 5th ed. Oxford: Oxford University Press, 2001.

Conclusion

In chapter one, we asked 'why bother with medical ethics?'. The first reason we gave was 'to pass exams'. This is an important reason. It explains the existence of the previous chapter and, let's face it, it might well be the reason why you purchased the book in the first place. In truth, it was *our* initial reason for writing this textbook! Our orders were clear: this new textbook should make sure that all medical students, even those who detest medical ethics, pass their ethics exams. We have done our best to meet this request.

But, beyond the immediate goal to guide students through the exam hoop, we had more ambitious aims. The first was to show that medical ethics is not the dry, boring subject that so many doctors and medical students think it is. In the right hands, it can nearly always be both intellectually challenging *and* entertaining. The second was to convince our readers that medical ethics could be useful in practice. Medical ethics has a role at the bedside, as well as in the meeting room of politicians. The Four Principles of medical ethics – Respect for Autonomy, Beneficence, Non-maleficence and Justice – deserve as much attention as the other 'famous four': Inspection, Palpation, Percussion and Auscultation. As we said in chapter one, the ethical and practical dimensions of medicine go hand in hand with each other.

Finally, perhaps the most far-fetched of our visions, we hoped that some readers might look back at the section on 'why bother with medical ethics?' and tut-tut in disappointment. "They got the order all wrong", they might say, "the most important reason for studying medical ethics is *not* to pass exams but, quite simply, to be a better doctor!".

At the very least, we have given you the facts and principles you require to practise medicine in a legal and ethical manner. Yet, however well you may know the criteria for assessing competence, the ethical issues relating to confidentiality, or the importance of human rights to medicine, this knowledge alone will not make you an ethical doctor – as someone once said, "that is your own affair".

Appendix A

The core curriculum for medical ethics and law[1]

1. Informed consent and refusal of treatment
- Why respect for autonomy is so important
- Adequate information
- Treatment without consent
- Competence
- Battery and negligence

2. The clinical relationship – truthfulness, trust and good communication
- Ethical limits of paternalism
- Building trust
- Honesty, courage and other virtues in clinical practice
- Narrative and the importance of communication skills

3. Confidentiality
- Clinical importance of privacy
- Compulsory and discretionary disclosure
- Public versus private interests

4. Medical research
- Ethical and legal tensions in doing medical research on patients, human volunteers, and animals
- The need for effective regulation

5. Human reproduction
- Ethical and legal status of the embryo/fetus
- Assisted conception
- Abortion
- Prenatal screening

6. The new genetics
- Treating the abnormal versus improving the normal
- Debates about the ethical boundaries of and the need to regulate genetic therapy and research

7. Children
- Ethical and clinical significance of age of consent to treatment
- Dealing with parental/child/clinician conflicts

8. Mental disorders and disabilities
- Ethical and legal justifications for detention and treatment without consent
- Conflicts of interests between patient, family and community

9. Life, death, dying and killing
- The duty of care and ethical and legal justification for the non-provision of life prolonging treatment and the provision of potentially life shortening palliatives
- Transplantation
- Death certification and the role of the coroner's court

10. Vulnerabilities created by the duties of doctors and medical students
- Public expectations of medicine
- The need for teamwork
- The health of doctors and students in relation to professional performance
- The GMC and professional regulation
- Responding appropriately to clinical mistakes
- Whistleblowing

11. Resource allocation
- Ethical debates about 'rationing' and the fair and just distribution of scarce health resources
- The relevance of needs, rights, utility, efficiency, merit and autonomy to theories of equitable health care
- Boundaries of responsibility of individuals for their own health

12. Rights
- What rights are, and their links with moral and professional duties
- The importance of the concept of rights, including human rights, for good medical practice.

References
1. British Medical Association; Medical Ethics Today. London: BMJ Publishing Group, 2004, 654-655.

Appendix B

How to get struck off

The General Medical Council receives thousands of complaints from dissatisfied patients and members of the public each year. As you can see from the table below, the number of complaints has increased considerably over the last 10 years.

Year	Total number of complaints
1995	1503
1996	2214
1997	2687
1998	3066
1999	3001
2000	4470
2001	4504
2002	3943

If a doctor is proved guilty, the GMC can:

• erase the doctor from the register.

• suspend the doctor's registration.

• place conditions on the doctor's registration.

• warn the doctor publicly but without affecting his registration.

In 2000, for example, 22% of the doctors charged with serious professional misconduct were judged not guilty by the GMC's Professional Conduct Committee, while 32% were struck off the register. The others were either suspended, reprimanded or given conditions on their registration.

How can I get struck off?

There are many, many ways to get struck off. The GMC kindly provided us with the most common reasons for erasing doctors from the register.

* Treatment without consent.

* Altering or not making adequate records.

* Inadequate or inappropriate treatment.

* Breach of confidentiality.

* Indecent behaviour towards patients or colleagues.

* Ignoring your professional responsibilities to your patients.

* False claim to qualifications or experience.

* Financial dishonesty.

* Other dishonesty, including theft.

* Irresponsible prescribing.

* Improper signing of certificate.

* Improper emotional or sexual relations with patients or colleagues.

* Misuse of drugs (including personal use and possession of drugs).

* Fraudulent research results.

* Improper delegation.

* Practising when a carrier of infectious disease.

Note: The hearings of the Professional Conduct Committee are public. The press are therefore invited to attend!

How to make unethical decisions

- Believe that medical ethics is irrelevant to medical practice.

- Believe that the Four Principles are:
  1. Non-beneficence
  2. Maleficence
  3. Respect for astronomy
  4. Injustice

- Believe that the dictum 'doctor knows best' is true in all cases.

- Make hurried decisions based on gut feeling without using your nut.

- Refuse to ask the advice of others.

Appendix C

Useful terms and conditions

Acts/omissions distinction – states that there may be a moral difference between actively doing something and omitting to do something, even if both result in the same consequences.

Ad hominem **fallacy** – criticising a person rather than his argument.

Advance directive – a type of advance statement, indicating that a person does not want to be treated in certain circumstances. Legally binding if certain conditions are met.

Appeal to authority – saying something is right because an authority says so.

Autonomy – refers to people's ability to make rational choices based on their own beliefs and values, free from the controlling influence of others.

Balancing – choosing which of two or more moral norms takes precedence over the other.

Battery – intentionally touching or injuring another person without his consent.

Beneficence (Principle of) – the obligation to provide net benefit to patients.

Best interests – an assessment of what is best for a person. Difficult to define. Varies from patient to patient. Depends in part on the patient's personal values and beliefs.

Bolam test – a test to determine whether a doctor breached an adequate standard of care. To pass the test, the doctor must have acted in accordance with a 'responsible body of medical opinion'.

Common law (or case law) – laws derived from the judgements of past cases. Sets out laws not covered in Acts of Parliament. In contrast to 'statute law', which consists of all the Acts passed by Parliament (e.g. the Mental Health Act or the Family Law Reform Act).

Competence – whether a patient is mentally or physically well enough to make an informed decision. Is task-specific.

Confidentiality – keeping your patients' secrets, or protecting a patient's personal information from unauthorised parties.

Consent – a patient's valid agreement to be treated.

Consequentialism – holds that an act is right or wrong depending solely on its consequences.

Deontology – holds that an act is right or wrong depending on whether it adheres to certain rules or principles.

DN(A)R order – DNR stands for 'Do Not Resuscitate'. Indicates that doctors should not attempt to revive a patient whose heart has just stopped beating.

Double Effect (Doctrine of) – permits an act that may have a bad effect if the intention is to bring about a good effect. The conditions are: that the intention is to bring about the good effect and not the bad effect (although it may be foreseen), that the good effect outweighs the bad effect, that the good effect actually is good, and that achieving the good effect does not depend on the bad effect occurring.

Ethics – hard to define. Simply, the study of morality and the moral life. Medical ethics is the study of the moral issues in medicine.

Euthanasia – deliberately killing a person – or allowing a person to die – as part of their medical treatment. Divided into active (positive intervention to kill), passive (omission to provide treatment allowing death), voluntary (the patient asks to die), non-voluntary (person is incompetent) and involuntary (person is competent and does not give consent to be killed).

Family Law Reform Act (1969) – states that competent children over 16 can consent to any treatment, even without the parents' consent.

Formula of Universal Law – a formulation of Kant's Categorical Imperative. States that you should 'act only on that maxim through which you can at the same time will that it should become a universal law'.

Formula of Humanity – another formulation of the Categorical Imperative. States that you should 'always treat people as ends and never merely as a means'.

Gillick competence – refers to a child under 16 who can consent to treatment by virtue of his intelligence and understanding of the proposed treatment.

Gradualist position (on abortion) – holds that the fetus acquires higher moral status as it develops in the womb. Our moral duties to the fetus therefore evolve as the pregnancy progresses.

Inductive fallacy of overgeneralization – making a broad generalisation from a small sample.

Justice – difficult to define. Different kinds exist: distributive, retributive, rights-based, legal, personal, social, etc. Crudely, giving people their fair share and not discriminating unfairly.

Kant – German footballer. Also, 18th century German philosopher who postulated the Categorical Imperative.

Kevin the Consequentialist – rude consequentialist hypochondriac with an unsightly mole on his face.

Logical fallacy – a mistake in the logical relation between a conclusion and its premises.

Mental Health Act – Act relevant to patients with mental disorders. In certain circumstances, allows doctors to override a mentally disabled patient's refusal of treatment and to forcibly restrain mentally disabled patients.

Moral status – protective concept preventing us from treating things in any way we like. Warren has suggested 7 principles of moral status: respect for life, anti-cruelty, agent's rights, human rights, ecological, interspecific, and transitivity of respect (see chapter 6).

Negligence – breach of a doctor's duty of care by providing a sub-standard level of care and causing the patient harm.

Non-maleficence (Principle of) – the obligation to avoid causing net harm.

Notifiable disease – one of dozens of diseases which a doctor is legally required to notify to a local authority, even if this breaches patient confidentiality.

No-true-Scotsman fallacy – rejecting a good counterargument by shifting the meaning of words.

'Ordinary versus extraordinary means' distinction – claims that it is morally acceptable to forgo extraordinary treatments but it is not acceptable to forgo ordinary treatments.

Osler, William – an excellent doctor, whose work should be read by all medics.

Paternalism – the deliberate overriding or non-consultation of a patient's wishes with the intention of benefiting the patient or avoiding him harm.

Person – being with high moral status to which we have the moral obligations we owe each other.

PRHO – stands for 'pre-registration house officer'. A newly qualified doctor.

Prima facie (principle) – a principle that is binding unless it conflicts with another prima facie principle.

Principlism (also known as the Four Principles approach) – holds that there are four, universally accepted moral principles that can be used to examine medico-ethical questions.

Proxy – a person who makes a decision on behalf of someone else.

Proxy consent – consent on behalf of a patient who cannot give consent himself. Consent on behalf of adults is not permitted in the United Kingdom. Parents may consent on behalf of children.

QALY (Quality Adjusted Life Year) – QALYs are used as a way of numerically scoring the outcomes of treatments to help us compare the overall benefits of different treatment options.

Rights – a form of entitlement stemming from moral, social, political or legal rules. Can be divided into 'legal' and 'moral' rights, and 'claim' and 'liberty' rights. Entail the existence of related duties (e.g. right to life ? duty not to kill).

Sesquipedalian – having many syllables (e.g. polysyllabic).

Slippery slope argument – if you allow A, which is at the top of the slope, you'll slide all the way down to E. There are two types: logical (where there are logical steps from A to E) and empirical (where the steps to the bottom are based on empirical assertions).

Specification – 'filling in' moral norms or principles in the light of specific cases to give them action-guiding content.

Statute law – the laws set out in Acts of Parliament. In contrast to common law, which is derived from the judgements of past cases.

Utilitarianism – a consequentialist moral theory that states that the right action is one that brings about the most utility. Utilitarians define 'utility' in different ways. For some, utility amounts to pleasure (hedonistic utilitarianism), for others it is satisfying people's wishes (preference utilitarianism) and for others still it is a combination of desirable things, such as beauty, love, friendship, pleasure and so on (pluralistic utilitarianism).

Virtue – many definitions exist. Here is a common one: a virtue is a character trait that promotes human flourishing.

Virtue theory – a theory that states that an action is right if it is what a virtuous person would characteristically do in the circumstances.

Yuk – expression of disgust. Is not a sufficient reason to condemn a practice. Must be supported by good reasons.

Appendix D

Useful contacts and resources

Medical Ethics Department
British Medical Association
BMA House
Tavistock Square
London WC1H 9JP
Tel: 0207 383 6286
E-mail: ethics@bma.org.uk
Website: www.bma.org.uk/ethics

Department of Health (UK)
Richmond House
79 Whitehall
London SW1A 2NS
Tel: 0207 210 4850
E-mail: dhmail@doh.gsi.gov.uk
Website: www.doh.gov.uk/index/html

Driver and Vehicle Licensing Agency (DVLA)
Drivers Medical Group
DVLA
Swansea SA99 1DL
Tel: 0870 600 0301
E-mail: eftd@dvla.gsi.gov.uk
Website: www.dvla.gov.uk

General Medical Council
178 Great Portland Street
London W1W 5JE
Tel: 0207 580 7642
E-mail: standards@gmc-uk.org
Website: www.gmc-uk.org

Human Fertilisation and Embryology Authority (HFEA)
Paxton House
30 Artillery Lane
London E1 7LS
Tel: 0207 377 5077
E-mail: admin@hfea.gov.uk
Website: www.hfea.gov.uk

Health Service Ombudsman (UK)
Tel: 0845 015 4033 or 0207 217 4163
E-mail: OHSC.Enquiries@ombudsman.gsi.gov.uk
Website: www.ombudsman.org.uk
The Ombudsman, who is independent of the NHS and the government, looks mainly into patient complaints about the NHS.

Medical and Dental Defence Union of Scotland
Mackintosh House
120 Blythswood Street
Glasgow G2 4EA
Tel: 0141 221 5858
E-mail: info@mddus.com
Website: www.mddus.com

Medical Defence Union
230 Blackfriars Road
London SE1 8JP
Tel: 0207 202 1500
E-mail: mdu@the-mdu.com
Website: www.the-mdu.com

Medical Protection Society
Granary Whark House
Leeds LS11 5PY
Tel: 0845 605 4000
E-mail: mpsmarketing@mps.org.uk
Website: www.mps.org.uk

National Patient Safety Agency
4-8 Maple Street
London W1T 5HD
Tel: 0207 927 9500
Website: www.npsa.nhs.uk

Royal College of Physicians of London
11 St. Andrews Place
Regent's Park
London NW1 4LE
Tel: 0207 487 5218
Website: www.rcplondon.ac.uk

World Medical Association
13 Chemin du Levant
CIB, Bâtiment A
01210 Ferney-Voltaire
France
Tel: +33 4 50 40 75 75
E-mail: wma@wma.net
Website: www.wma.net

Our Favourites...

Medical ethics journals
* Journal of Medical Ethics (www.jmedethics.com)
* Journal of Medicine and Philosophy (www.szp.swets.nl)
* Cambridge Quarterly of Healthcare Ethics (http://titles.cambridge.org/journals)

Other medical ethics textbooks
* Hope T, Savulescu J, Hendrick J. *Medical ethics and law; the core curriculum.* London: Churchill Livingstone, 2003. (£15.99)
  Comments: Has an appealing layout with boxes and bullet points and lots of subheadings for clarity and ease of reference. Good list of references at the end of each chapter.

* Gillon R. *Philosophical medical ethics.* Chichester: John Wiley & Sons, 1985. (£37.50)
  Comments: Although slightly dated, it is still one of the most readable and enjoyable books on medical ethics on the market.

* Beauchamp T, Childress J. *Principles of Biomedical Ethics.* 5th ed. Oxford: Oxford University Press, 2001. (£22.95)
  Comments: A comprehensive look at many aspects of medical ethics. More advanced than the other books in this section. Has an interesting description and discussion of important cases in medical ethics at the end.

* British Medical Association; **Medical Ethics Today.** London: BMJ Publishing Group, 2004. (£60)
  Comments: A huge, expensive book that covers a vast area of medical ethics. A superb reference work. Includes a searchable CD ROM of the book.

Introductions to ethics and moral philosophy

- Raphael DD. *Moral philosophy.* Second ed. Oxford: Oxford University Press, 1994. (£13.99)
  Comments: Very short, clear, and – most importantly – interesting. The second edition includes a new chapter on medical ethics.

- Rachels J. *The elements of moral philosophy.* Second ed. Englewood Cliffs: Prentice-Hall, 1993. (£23.99)
  Comments: Lively and nicely written, covers the basic of moral theory and addresses topics such as famine relief and the treatment of animals.

- Benn P. *Ethics.* London: Routledge, 1998. (£16)
  Comments: Covers a lot of ground. Explains difficult concepts in non-technical language and with occasional touches of humour.

Medical ethics and law websites

- **UK Clinical Ethics Network** (www.ethics-network.org.uk)
  Comments: An Oxford-based website targetted at clinical ethics committees, but with lots of information of potential interest to doctors and medical students. Includes a useful section detailing the policies and guidelines of the GMC, BMA and other organisations on a range of issues from consent to resource allocation.

- **Her Majesty's Stationary Office** (www.hmso.gov.uk)
  Comments: An easy-to-navigate website with searchable UK legislation since 1988.

- **Bioethics.net** (www.bioethics.net)
  Comments: Has regular updates on medical ethics news and introductions to many medical ethics topics. It is also the website of the American Journal of Bioethics.

- **Breaking Bioethics News** (http://msnbc.msn.com/id/3035344)
  Comments: Interesting commentaries on topical issues in medical ethics by two respected ethicists.

- **Philosophy Radio** (www.angelfire.com/ego/philosophyradio)
  Comments: Excellent website with recordings of radio programmes on philosophy, including medical ethics.

Books on being a doctor (ideal for holidays)

* Kaplan J. *The dressing station; a surgeon's odyssey.* Chatham: Picador, 2002. (£6.99)
  Comments: A doctor, who refuses the comforts of working in a well-equipped hospital, travels all over the world practising medicine in terrible and unusual places. Gripping stuff.

* Gawande, A. *Complications; a surgeon's notes on an imperfect science.* London: Profile Books Ltd, 2002. (£7.99)
  Comments: Musings of a literate surgeon on the art of medicine and a life spent cutting people up. Includes a chilling chapter on necrotising fasciitis. Do not read before meals.

* Peters CJ and Olshaker M. *Virus Hunter.* New York: Anchor Books, 1998. (£7.99)
  Comments: CJ Peters, ex-Chief of Special Pathogens at the Centers for Disease Control in the United States, recounts 30 years of travelling around the world chasing 'hot' viruses (including Ebola!). Fascinating and entertaining.

Acknowledgements

Writing this textbook has been a monumental task. When we accepted the job, neither of us quite knew how many late nights would be spent working on yet another draft! We dread to think how we would have coped without the help of the dozens of people who generously gave us their time, support and expertise.

The most substantial contribution has come from Catherine Quarini, currently a 4th year medical student, who wrote much of chapter 10. We cannot thank her enough for her excellent work.

Professor Raanan Gillon kindly accepted to write the Foreword. His influence on the book will be apparent to many. Dr Piers Benn cast an unforgiving, philosophical eye over the chapter on moral theory. The chapter on medical research (chapter 5) was greatly enriched by the astute comments of Dr Richard Ashcroft. Jo Bridgeman checked over the chapter on children (chapter 8) and did much to improve the accuracy of the text. Dr Huw Dorkins gave extremely useful insights into his work as a clinical geneticist and provided helpful comments on chapter 7. The excellent advice and feedback of Dr Phil Davison, a consultant psychiatrist, refined the chapter on mental disorders (chapter 9). Ronald P. Sokol, an esteemed lawyer and legal philosopher, patiently shared many hours explaining the intricacies of the law and shaped the chapter on rights (chapter 13). Professor Jonathan Montgomery contributed a helpful account of the relevance of the Human Rights Act to doctors in the UK to that same chapter. Dr Sonya Babu-Narayan, a cardiology registrar, contributed a useful section on 'coalface ethics and the junior doctor' (chapter 11).

Catriona Richardson and Dr Stephanie Bown, of the Medical Protection Society, sent us a wealth of information regarding consent and confidentiality in addition to much appreciated feedback. Kate Walmsley, of the General Medical Council, did a considerable amount of research to provide us with relevant GMC statistics and a list of common reasons for getting struck off from the register (Appendix B). Dr Mike Parker, Dr Nafsika Athanassoulis, Dr Christopher Cowley, Dr Richard Ashcroft and Dr Martin von Fragstein have all shared their 'tips from the top' in the chapter on 'passing exams' (chapter 14). Various doctors, patients and medical students have shared their experiences with us and given us permission to reproduce their stories in the book, albeit anonymously. To all those above, we are incredibly grateful. The book has benefited much from your contributions.

We would also like to thank the many doctors, philosophers, and medical students, who read over chapters of the book and offered their perceptive comments on early drafts: Katherine MacDonald, Diego Silva, Anna Smajdor, Chris Hourigan, Matthew Sydes, Helen Corke, Sharon Cuthbert, Matthew Rogers, John Whitaker, Mara Cohn, Tamara Curtin, Trudi Foreman, Justin Cramer, Tim Cominos, Ilene Lewis, Lee Barash, Annette Weil, Michael Buckley, Anna Gaskell, Rachel Ives, Louisa Beringer, Emily Ferenczi, Suzanne Gill, Alison Hook, Katherine Richards, Emma Rhodes and Caroline Whitwood.

A special thanks must be made to Dr Christopher Cowley, Lecturer in Medical Ethics, University of East Anglia Medical School, for the hours he spent reviewing our draft copy and for his many suggestions.

We are grateful to our superb cartoonists, Nigel Sutherland, Nick Kim, Hemant Morparia and Sydney Harris, whose hilarious cartoons provide much needed relief throughout the book.

Daniel would like to thank his mother and father, André, Georges, Charlie and Sam for their patience and moral support. They dragged me away from my desk and stoically endured many tedious conversations about the book. If death by boredom was possible, they would not be here today.

Gill would like to thank her family and friends who have helped with this project in numerous ways. Special thanks to Mum for all the proof-reading, often at very short notice, and to Rachel for your excellent comments. To Mum, Dad, Ian and John for being there, and for reminding me how to have fun! Thanks to everyone on firm 2, to all at Littlemore, and to anyone else I have forgotten to mention. Finally, thanks to Matt for all your patience and support over the last few months.

Finally, we are both indebted to our excellent editor, Ashley McKimm, for his enthusiasm and constant willingness to help.

Oxford, January 2005

D.K.S.
G.B.

Index

Buying this book

Thanks to the unique way in which trauma is funded each book in the series helps to support a different charity. It means you can feel good in the knowledge that buying this book makes a small contribution to help something big happen for the better.

This book supports the important work of Médecins Sans Frontières (MSF). Here's what you'll be helping …

About Médecins Sans Frontières

MSF is a leading non-governmental organization for emergency medical aid. We provide independent medical relief to victims of war, disasters and epidemics in over 80 countries around the world, treating those who need it most, regardless of ethnic origin, religion or political affiliation.

To get access to, and care for, the most vulnerable, MSF must remain scrupulously independent of governments, as well as religious and economic powers. We rely on private individuals for the majority of our funding.

In the field, we conduct our own assessments, manage projects directly and monitor the impact of our aid. MSF insists on exercising its responsibility to speak out when it sees that those we are trying to help are being abused. We campaign locally and internationally for greater respect for humanitarian law and the right of civilians to impartial humanitarian assistance. We also campaign for fairer access to medicines and health care for the world's poorest people.

MSF is a voluntary organization. Each year, about 3 000 doctors, nurses, logistics specialists and engineers of all nationalities leave on field assignments. They work closely with thousands of national staff.

If you're a medical student and want to know more about MSF go to:
http://www.uk2.msf.org/working4us/MedicalStudents.htm

For more general information on MSF visit:
www.uk.msf.org

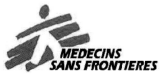

Guaranteed Pass

We've worked hard at trauma to produce the best Medical Ethics and Law textbook we can, and like all good textbooks should, we're willing to stand by it. We're so confident that you'll have a smooth passage through to graduation with our help that we'll give you your money back if you don't – simple as that.

It's the same with all books in the trauma Survival Guide series.

Obviously we can't guarantee that you'll pass end-of-firm exams or that lunchtime quiz every Friday. What we can promise is that if by chance, natural disaster or act of God you don't graduate fully from medical school with the help of our books we'll refund the cost in full.

We're confident that with a little motivation on your part we'll never need to prove this claim to you, however if you don't have as much faith as we do make sure you keep your receipt. You can request a claim form in this unlikely event via books@traumaroom.com.

Good luck (not that we expect you to need it).

Please view the full terms and conditions available at www.traumaroom.com.